MW00378908

ROOT CAUSE

Turning Symptoms to Solutions

Christie Brooks, Functional Medicine, MS, RD, LD

Niche Pressworks

Root Cause: Turning Symptoms to Solutions

ISBN-13: 978-1-952654-28-2 Paperback
          978-1-952654-29-9 eBook

Copyright © 2021 by Christie Brooks, Functional Medicine Registered Dietitian

All rights reserved. No part of this book may be used or reproduced in any manner whatsoever without prior written consent of the author, except as provided by the United States of America copyright law.

This book is written as a source of information only. It is intended to provide helpful and informative material on the subjects addressed in the publication. The information contained in this book should by no means be considered a substitute for prescribed medicines by your qualified medical professional.

All efforts have been made to ensure the accuracy of the information contained in this book as of the date published.

Permission of copyright photo given by IFM (Institute of Functional Medicine), 2020.

For permission to reprint portions of this content or bulk purchases, contact Christie Brooks at www.ChristieBrooksRD.com.

Published by Niche Pressworks; http://NichePressworks.com.

Dedication

To the utterance "your labs are ok, so you are ok" and the relentless fatigue, trauma, stress, and time you stole from my family, my life, and all the hard work you created...I dedicate this to you.

For you ignited an unsatiable fire—a hunger and thirst for biochemical knowledge, resulting in a new birth within me. You had to break me in order to make me...to rise up in fulfilling my purpose.

And to all my brothers and sisters who are suffering and searching for health answers, I pray that my journey, my hard work, will ignite your own fire, inspire your hope, and give you answers for your own unique journeys.

Contents

Dedication..iii

Introduction ix

The End of My Rope Was the Beginning ix

The Typical Healthcare Route Had No Answers x

Taking Stock of My Situation xi

I. Was. Finally. Heard...xi

Finding Solutions..xii

Passing on What I Now Know xiii

Chapter 1: You're Not Crazy...1

Your Unique Journey: Listening to the Symptoms, Not Just Labs 1

Patients Like You Have Found Answers...2

Your Health Is a Tapestry Woven of Mind, Body, and Spirit................8

Chapter 2: The Medical Industry is Upside Down....................11

Money-Driven Medicine..11

You Have More Control Than You Think 12

7 Reasons Why You Should Get Started Now 13

Chapter 3: Take Control of Your Health......................................17

Hidden Lifestyle Costs of Being Unhealthy....................................17

Your Health: Questionnaire 18

It Doesn't Have to Be This Way: Taking Charge of Your Health 23

How Much Does It Cost to Do Small Daily Changes? 23

8 Myths We Need to Bust..25

Take Heart from Others' Success...28

Ready to Learn More? 31

Chapter 4:   How Functional Medicine Works 33

Getting to Root Causes 33

Functional Medicine Can Help 35

Mind-Body-Spirit—All Affect Each Other 36

Who Practices Functional Medicine? 39

The Functional Medicine Tree Perspective 39

Alternative Healing as Complement, Not Competitor 40

Chapter 5:   A Major Health Culprit: Stress 43

Are You "Running from a Bear"? 43

The Autonomic Nervous System 45

Common Characteristics of People Living in Chronic Stress Mode and Sympathetic Dominance: 47

Living in Chronic Stress and Sympathetic Dominance 47

How to Correct Sympathetic Dominance from Chronic Stress..........48

Chapter 6:   HPA Axis, Adrenal Dysfunction, and Issues..................51

Are You an Overwhelmed Baker? 51

The Endocrine Pyramid: Root Cause Healing from Ground Up 52

The Complexity of the Endocrine System 53

Cortisol Effects on Blood Sugar:
Weight Gain and Metabolic Syndrome..........................55

Did you know? 56

Middle Tier: The Thyroid 56

So, Is Your Root Cause Diagnosis HPA-Axis Adrenal Dysfunction? 62

Six Natural Ways to Improve Energy 62

Chapter 7:   Digestive Issues 65

If You Want to Fix Your Health, Start with Your Gut..........65

Your "Second Brain" 66

Questionnaire: How's Your Digestive System?................................67

Stress on the HPG Axis 69

Tips for Healing Your Gut: A Holistic Functional Medicine Approach 71

Chapter 8: **Inflammation—More Common than You Think** 75

Are you curious whether you have inflammation? See if you have any
of these issues: 76

Food Plays a Major Role in Inflammation 78

How to Fight Inflammation 79

Other Ways to Fight Inflammation (Reduce Oxidative Stress):..........80

More Food Tips 83

Chapter 9: **Sleep—A Foundational Solution** 85

What Sleep Does for Your Health 86

Sleep Reboots Hormones, Metabolism, Nervous System 87

Processes of Sleep: Circadian Rhythms 87

How Much Sleep Do We Need? 88

Tips for Better-Quality Sleep 88

Chapter 10: **Overcoming Obstacles** 93

What Matters Most? 93

Old Childhood Habits: "I Was Made to Clean My Plate" 94

"I Can't Afford the Money/Time" 94

Being Unhealthy Costs More Money than You Realize 96

"I Want Quicker Results." 98

"My Family Will Never Do Things This New Way"..........................100

"I Can Never Be/Do [Insert Comparison Here]." 101

"But My Willpower Failed Me in the Past!" 103

Budget Shopping 103

My Favorite Insider Shopping Hacks 105

Chapter 11: The Power of Holistic Focus 107

    Spirit and Mind: When the "Ah-Ha" Moment Strikes 107

    Healing and Self-Discovery 110

    Tips for Listening to Your "Guiding Power" 111

    A New Script 112

Chapter 12: Get the Most from Your Consultation 115

    What Next? 115

    My Areas of Specialty 115

    What You Can Expect from Treatment 116

    You Don't Have to Be Local—I Offer Telemedicine 117

    Planning Your First Visit 118

    What to Have Before We Start 120

    When You're Ready to Get Started 120

Thank You 123

Acknowledgments 125

About the Author 127

Introduction

The End of My Rope Was the Beginning

I was so tired that my tired was tired.

Exhaustion pierced into every cell of my being. Don't get me wrong—I've had days where I needed a cup of coffee to kick start a productive day, but THIS...THIS was not average tiredness. This was so different. It was a debilitating fatigue and an elevation of exhaustion I had never experienced. I felt the weight of the impossible crushing me. My brain refused sleep at 2:12 a.m. At some moments, my heart was racing so rapidly that I couldn't breathe. For the first time ever, I started experiencing anxiety and panic attacks. If you've never had those, and all of a sudden, they punch you in the face, the experience will absolutely terrify you!

I'm a mom of two very active kids. I HAD to live on the go. But my body was refusing every effort I could squander up. Before, I'd always been a people person, a people pleaser, and a helper, and I loved large gatherings with friends. But now, for some strange reason, I became fearful and anxious of being in crowds—even small ones. Small things would send me into uncontrollable crying frenzies; I'd become an emotional wreck for no reason. A deep, dark cloud of depression became my new shadow. I was worn out from trying, striving. The emotional demands kept bringing relentless fatigue, stress, hormonal strains, and burnout.

Almost overnight, I became an emotional and physical basket case, and I couldn't understand how I, the type A extrovert, had even gotten there.

I would have paid my life's savings for someone to get my kids up and ready for school. My body was physically present, but my brain fog did not allow me to be fully "present" with my family or work. Everything was a blur. Work was almost impossible.

Who would have thought putting a load of laundry in the washer would be so daunting? Just stopping to get milk felt as if I had run a marathon. Twelve hours of sleep were never enough, yet I could not fall asleep at night because my mind ran races that never seemed to have a finish line.

The eye-opener came when I forgot to pick up my kids from school because my brain fog had me on lockdown. Now, WHO DOES THAT? I got the Mom Fail Card that day!

THIS is where I was. But this is not who I am.

I found myself on the ground, covered in sloppy tears, crying out to God in despair. My rope only had a few threads left. I was losing it.

The Typical Healthcare Route Had No Answers

"Your lab tests are completely ok. There's nothing wrong with you. We just need to put on you on depression medicine." This was the general news I got from the several doctors I saw.

How could they say there was nothing wrong with me?

I felt as if they were talking to me like I was crazy...as if I had lost my mind. If something similar has happened to you, maybe you are feeling me here?

I may have looked perfectly fine on the outside, but I was a broken-down train wreck on the inside. Without proper lab work to prove what was taking place, the conventional medicine route left me feeling lost and alone. I even doubted my own feelings that something was physically wrong! Maybe I *was* depressed, as the doctors said. Maybe it *was* all in my head, as they inferred.

But I couldn't accept that diagnosis. I knew without a doubt that something was going on in my body that they weren't seeing.

I. Knew. It.

Taking Stock of My Situation

Let's back up. I didn't get here overnight.

My current situation had come from a slow progression and buildup of many stressful or grieving events in my forty-plus years on this earth. Being a type A personality, I had a drive for perfection. I had no time for self-care because I was always putting others first without establishing personal boundaries.

I put an insane amount of pressure on myself, believing I could easily conquer an absurd daily to-do list. I was a soccer mom, homeroom mom, wife, and career woman—and I still had dinner cooked every night and laundry washed and put up after I did my hour of daily exercise. I was an expert at juggling. I just managed what life threw at me.

Or so I thought. In reality, I had been struggling and striving to keep my head above water for a long time. And now, I was at my wit's end. And after hearing the same thing from multiple doctors, I had given up.

But something within still resisted the idea that I was physically "fine," as they kept telling me.

I. Was. Finally. Heard.

Around the time when I was totally at a loss for what to do next, I had a regular checkup with my OBGYN nurse practitioner, T.J. Moix. She mentioned something that opened the door for me to tell her my struggles... and she actually listened. What she said next profoundly affected me—it was as if the world stopped to listen, and my eyes welled up with tears. She said that it sounded like I had Hypothalamus-Pituitary-Adrenal (HPA) Axis Dysfunction, or Adrenal Dysfunction.

This disorder results from an accumulation of stress and/or trauma over a period of years. Urine tests could confirm it, but a four-point saliva cortisol test would give me a way to capture my cortisol pattern in a day, and a six-point would give me a cortisol awakening response along with the cortisol pattern for the day.

A saliva cortisol test? No other doctor had ever mentioned this type of test to me so that I could see my production (or lack thereof) pattern!

Finally, someone had HEARD me. For the first time in a LONG time, I felt a glimmer of hope.

In fact, T.J. had had her own struggles with HPA-Axis Adrenal Dysfunction, and she had also encountered several frustrating situations with patients who were doing everything at 100 percent but were still not losing weight. She knew she was missing something that her conventional/Western medicine training was not providing. (This reminded me of similar frustrations about situations in which my clients weren't losing weight after being 100 percent on a calorie-controlled diet!) Without a doubt, the Lord led me to T.J. because her quest for answers was also my answer.

To this day, I'm forever thankful for her openness and direction that she discovered. She gave me HOPE. Are you hearing me? HOPE!

Finding Solutions

I went through saliva testing to test my cortisol, and the diagnosis came in: Yes, HPA-Axis Adrenal Dysfunction was the problem.

Why did it take so long to learn this? Why hadn't they done this testing before? Why hadn't I known?

My medical training was not quite up to speed in finding the solutions to my symptoms.

Pharmacists Kelly Stanley and Kelly Wilkins at Stanley Compounding Center interpreted my saliva testing and set me in the direction of temporary hormone replacement. Their help, along with lots and lots of related research studies, began my healing journey. I used a combination of diet adjustments, healing supplements, temporary hormone replacement therapy, a new exercise plan, and temporary supplemental hormone therapy to heal my body.

On days I was too debilitated to do much but spend time alone with God, I grew closer in relationship with Him. My self-awareness surged. I became more aware of my emotions and of my breathing patterns. I felt an indescribable sense of peace being born within me. While my body was healing, these moments showed that my mind and spirit were healing, too.

In hindsight, the Lord was growing me in knowledge in all those areas—mind, body, and spirit. It was as if He was preparing me for what was to come...bringing me to where I am now so that my suffering would not be in vain, but it would be for me to help others. He transformed a dark situation into something beautiful. The connection of Mind-Body-Spirit was not just something I read about; I experienced it in raw, living form. It transformed my beliefs on healing and opened my eyes to see what I had been fooled about for years.

As I shared my story with others regarding my frustration and struggle searching for answers (only to hit roadblocks) and finally getting answers and healing through Functional Medicine, people—mostly women—started reaching out. They had similar symptoms and were not getting answers from the typical healthcare route. That fact, along with helping my daughter struggle with health issues of her own since the age of twelve, eventually led me to advance my education and become a Functional Medicine Registered Dietitian.

Passing on What I Now Know

If you have arrived at this point in your journey and still don't have answers as to how to regain your life back, my hope is to give you that "ah-ha" moment and reassure you that you are not alone in your struggles and that there is definite hope. My own quest to heal my mind, body, and spirit was a long one, and many times I found myself on dead-end roads without answers. But eventually, I found those answers—and you can, too.

For more than twenty-five years, I've specialized in helping people like you. It is time we turn medical symptoms into solutions instead of just taking medicine after medicine for the rest of our lives, since that is only putting a bandage on the real problem.

While my issue was Adrenal Dysfunction, yours could be any number of things. And if you're frustrated and discouraged and feel you can't find answers, I feel you. You've come to the right place.

- What if you could get off all those medicines and get to a comfortable weight you are proud of?

  Just imagine how you would feel to notice your stamina, libido, and energy level coming back.

- What would it feel like to be free of fatigue, brain fog, overstimulation, and that overwhelming feeling of stress?

- What would it be like to be healthy again?

- You're about to find out.

But first, let's take a look at why the answers have been so hard to get through conventional methods.

CHAPTER 1

You're Not Crazy

If everyone is telling you that you are "fine," that your labs are okay so you are okay, shouldn't you believe them?

Not necessarily.

Our knowledge of our own bodies goes way deeper than limited tests can go. When we have body awareness, we know when something is a little "off." Just because our blood labs might be a "low normal" or "high normal" does not confirm we are "ok."

Your Unique Journey: Listening to the Symptoms, Not Just Labs

Trying to fit yourself into the cookie-cutter diagnosis and treatment protocol of common healthcare doesn't always make sense, especially since your own situation—and biochemistry—is unique, as are the causes of your symptoms.

Functional Medicine does NOT rely only on labs to tell you when something's wrong or to just "manage" your symptoms and disease with more drugs; but instead, Functional Medicine practitioners use symptoms, dives into Mind-Body-Spirit past and present, and tighter lab ranges to help diagnose and treat the real cause. In more complex situations, multiple causes may be contributing, which is another reason why cookie-cutter protocols don't work. Sometimes prescription drugs are inevitable, but it is essential to address the root cause as well as to wean off those drugs if at all possible.

It's important to know the whole picture, not just a few pieces to the health puzzle. For example, the most commonly ordered labs for determining thyroid health don't provide the full picture of the thyroid. In addition, multiple other factors can affect thyroid function (see chapter 6), so merely looking at these already incomplete labs doesn't give a whole picture at all.

It's imperative that practitioners look at symptoms instead of just cookie-cutter labs that insurance only pays. And it's essential to dive into all aspects, upstream and downstream, of Mind-Body-Spirit to get the answers. You are not crazy!

Patients Like You Have Found Answers

Here are some examples of clients whose lab tests showed they were "okay" but who knew they weren't. They kept searching, and eventually, they found healing instead of disease management or dependency on meds.

Case #1: A Nervous System (HPA-Axis) Breakdown

"Susan" came to me as a forty-eight-year-old, slightly overweight mom of three active teens. Like most moms, she was always busy, and she also managed a farm during the day while her husband was out working. Susan was extremely fatigued and had gastrointestinal issues that went from constipation to diarrhea. She would have one good day, then be barely able to function for the next week or two, and her symptoms didn't seem prompted by anything she was doing or eating.

Susan rated her stress level at a seven out of ten. However, after a thorough discussion with her, I learned that she had had some very serious rough patches in her marriage, and some of these issues were still surfacing, making it a ten-out-of-ten stress level. Her sleep and anxiety had worsened since the marriage issues began, and she had recently experienced frequent nightmares. After seeing multiple doctors over the past few years and being told it was "just mental" and "just stress," she came to me.

She voiced that her first priority was to start feeling better, and then she wanted to lose some of the weight she had recently gained.

Diagnosis: After lab review and our hour-and-a-half discussion, it was pretty clear Susan had multiple issues: candida, unhealthy gut microbiome, adrenal issues (Fight-or-Flight Mode cortisol and sympathetic nervous system issues), excessive estrogen, low progesterone, low testosterone, low dehydroepiandrosterone (DHEA), and inflammation through her whole body. Her thyroid labs showed she was on the edge of hypothyroidism.

Goals: We needed to address several things:

- Improve Susan's gut health

- Improve her thyroid function

- Calm the adrenal glands and nervous system

- Improve her sleep

- Improve body cell powerhouse functioning

- Heal the gut

- Decrease inflammation

Treatment: I put Susan on the following treatment regimen:

- Supplements to support her thyroid

- Nutraceuticals and vitamin support for the adrenal glands

- Short temporary trial of progesterone and testosterone compounded hormone replacement (I do this ONLY if my client wants immediate changes instead of giving it a month or so to feel better)

- For the nervous system, diaphragmatic breathing techniques to calm the anxiety, meditation for ten minutes a day, Christian reiki, and yoga (specifically trauma yoga)

- Encouragement to also see a mental health therapist

Three months later: Susan reported that she was starting to feel normal again, and her sleep and bathroom issues were no longer a problem. "I think that probiotic you put me on has really helped me," she said. "And though I thought meditation was a little weird, I took your advice, and now I listen to the guided meditation for ten minutes each day. I can really tell the difference when I skip it." In addition, Susan and her husband started seeing a mental health therapist to address their marriage issues. "It seems I'm more at ease and having less anxiety-like problems," she said.

Case #2: "Mark": Medicated "Type A" Workaholic

Mark was fifty-eight years old, married, and had no more children still living at home. He worked an extremely stressful job with long hours and drank five to seven cups of coffee each day. His wife suffered from poor health, so he took care of her a lot when he wasn't working, and he had little time to exercise. His sister had encouraged him to see me since he was in survival mode and exhausted. He averaged five to six hours of sleep per night, interrupted by the need to get up to urinate.

Diagnosis: Mark was forty-five pounds overweight, and his doctor had already diagnosed him with high blood pressure. He had blood sugars over 150 (70-110 is the preferred range) and HgbA1c at 9 percent. (Hemoglobin A1c is a three-month average of blood sugars. The preferred Functional Medicine range is 4-5.5 percent; Mark's was very high by comparison.) He had refused blood-pressure medicine. He told me his doctor had put him on metformin (diabetes medicine) to allow him to eat what he wanted whenever he wanted, despite his other issues. I'm sure this was not the doctor's motive; however, Mark "heard" it to mean he could eat anything he wanted as long as he took the pill. Mark told me he just wanted to lose weight so that he could avoid blood-pressure medicine.

Goals: We needed to address several issues.
- Get to the bottom of his desire to take medication: When someone thinks they can depend on medicine so they can eat whatever they want, it's usually either out of fear (of being overwhelmed by

4

changing their diet), or they really do not care (which means they need some education about the potential medication drawbacks)

- Decrease inflammation

- Decrease the amount of caffeine consumption

- Balance blood sugars

- Improve sleep

- Calm his nervous system

- Boost his mitochondria powerhouses in his cells

- Increase his stress resiliency

Treatment: During our consultation, I determined that Mark's issue regarding taking medication instead of changing his diet was mainly fear, which is very common. With that in mind, Mark and I went over the following treatment plan:

- A very simplified meal plan catered specifically to address his blood sugar and blood pressure issues, which Mark admitted would be easier to follow than he had presumed (This plan would also help address his nocturnal urination, which was due to his elevated blood sugars.)

- Cutting back on coffee and replacing it with water or hot tea

- Starting some daily movements like walking

- Taking supplements to calm the stress hormone and improve blood pressure and blood sugars

Three months later: Once Mark saw how simple the nutrition plan actually was, he had also become very open to trying other suggestions for improving sleep and cutting back on caffeine. In addition, Mark's wife also felt she would benefit from the nutrition regimen, making food preparation even easier for Mark. "Not only have my blood sugars and blood pressure improved, but my wife is improving her health as well. Honestly, I can't believe this," Mark said. "I guess you were right; food IS medicine. See, look at my belt. It is now two holes down because I've lost the extra weight. I feel very full, never feeling hungry, yet I've lost weight. Now that is crazy!" Mark was also able to sleep through the night without having to go to the bathroom due to his improved blood sugars. "I did take your advice and went back to my doctor regarding the blood pressure medicine," he reported. "He says I don't need it now! My blood pressure is now back to normal because of the changes I made. So, thank you! It feels good to feel good again."

Case Study #3: "Angie" with Extreme Anxiety

Angie's story was much like mine. When she came to me, she could not function normally, but her labs were normal. "I knew I might be off, but I felt like they were calling me crazy," she said. "I even started questioning myself if I was going crazy, but I knew my body was not normal. How I felt was not normal. I was losing hope."

Angie was sometimes so exhausted that she could not even get off the couch. She had irregular, mucus-filled bowel movements that only occurred around every three days and smelled foul. She felt dizzy and foggy-brained. She couldn't get rid of her anxiety and tremors. Her symptoms were worse around her period. She was only getting about three hours of sleep at a time each night and tried to sleep when she could during the day. "The best way to describe it is that my body is attacking itself," she said. One of her doctors had diagnosed her with Meniere's disease, and she had accepted that diagnosis yet still sought better treatment. Her tongue was completely covered in white, indicating candida (which explained the mucus and foul-smelling bowel movements). She also had a scalloped-shaped tongue, indicating inadequate nervous system rest and sleep.

Diagnosis: Angie's testing indicated that she had HPA-Axis Adrenal Dysfunction, much like my own situation had been, and questionable mold exposure.

Goals: Our goals for Angie included the following:
- Improve her cortisol awakening response

- Decrease elevated cortisol at night and restore proper functioning to the adrenal glands

- Improve the microbiome (lining) of the gut to kill off candida and replenish the good bacteria (This also included the increased proper production of neurotransmitters, specifically GABA for anxiety.)

- Shift her out of sympathetic dominance

- Replenish her nervous system, HPA Axis, and mitochondria with the necessary vitamins and minerals in which she was deficient

- Test for mold toxicity

Treatment:
- Adaptogens with proper raw adrenal for the morning and with phosphatidylserine with theanine at night

- Supplements to reinoculate gut health and kill off candida

- Tongue scraping first thing each morning

- Supplements to support mitochondria

- Guided meditation daily for fifteen minutes and diaphragmatic breathing four times daily

- An anti-inflammatory diet, including avoidance of gluten, dairy, and all caffeine

- Yoga at least three times a week, one being a one-on-one trauma yoga session

- Christian reiki

Three months later: After three months of treatment, her bowels had become normal. She had only had tremors and anxiety attacks once. She had more energy in the mornings and noted it took her less time to fall asleep at night. She was still fudging a little on the dairy but did well cutting out on gluten and caffeine. She had begun to look forward to her yoga and meditation, and she had found an app that reminded her to do the diaphragmatic breathing. "I definitely am better than I was," she told me. "I can't wait to be well all the way!"

Your Health Is a Tapestry Woven of Mind, Body, and Spirit

The previous case studies reflect completely different scenarios. Each person had extensive health symptoms that emerged from multiple life shifts in the past or present that affected mind, body, spirit.

Their doctors, in the limited amount of time they had with them, no doubt did what they knew to do in trying to figure out what was going on with them. However, due to their unwanted time constraints, they had likely not been able to explore the equally important aspects of their patients' stress and trauma histories—their minds and spirits.

These are some examples of the ways a Functional Medicine practitioner can partner with conventional medical providers for better results. I had the time to dig deeply into all aspects of each patient's mind, body, and spirit in order to compile a customized healing regimen for each of them that treated all aspects—mind, body, and spirit.

We are like tapestries, each uniquely woven through time by different colors of life experiences, food choices, lifestyle choices, and family health history. No two tapestries are alike, yet they are all woven with the same principles:

1. The interaction of multiple body systems

2. Hormones

3. Stress/Trauma

4. Sleep

5. Relationships/Community/Support

6. Movement

7. Breath

What this means is that though you and others may have similar health goals, the way you achieve them will differ. For example, if you want to lose weight but your hormonal balance is off, a cookie-cutter, twelve-hundred-calorie meal plan will most likely not help you. And when I say hormones, I'm not talking sex hormones only...I'm talking about all hormones: cortisol, cortisone, insulin, thyroid hormones, ghrelin, leptin, estrogen, progesterone, DHEA, testosterone, etc.

We need to look at your intricately made person, that Mind-Body-Spirit tapestry, from all angles and from its beginning to its current situation. In other words, we need to take a Functional Medicine approach.

It is possible to find your solutions—and when you really start thinking about what your poor health is doing to your life, the need to find them suddenly feels a lot more urgent.

CHAPTER 2

The Medical Industry is Upside Down

Money-Driven Medicine

Look, I am going to be totally upfront and direct with you in this short book because you've probably been around the block one too many times without getting the answers or the help you desperately crave.

The conventional medicine industry is a broken system. It's not that the doctors don't care...because they really do care. We all chose to be in the medical profession because we want to transform people's lives.

Unfortunately, in America, our system functions on three main principles, and they don't always serve in the best interest of the patient:

1. Insurance companies drive almost all care decisions for covered services.
   - They control how much a hospital gets paid for patient care and how much time that should take.
   - They control what procedures and labs are covered and which ones aren't.
   - They set and control what drugs they'll cover and at what price.

○ They charge you absurdly costly premiums, set the co-pay, and then lay a bunch of fees and restrictions on how you use the money YOU have been paying them.

○ They will not pay a claim if it is out of their approved network, within which they've made cost agreements with certain doctors.

2. If a hospital or a clinic wants to offer insurance-covered care, they are at the mercy of the insurance companies' guidelines.

3. Doctors are under immense pressure to see more patients in less time to keep the hospital or clinic profitable. To keep on schedule, they often have to suggest you do your own research or refer you to outside resources. (This is where I can help.)

Let me give you an example. "Marsha" came to me wanting to get off her type 2 diabetes medication. Her doctor had her on prescription medication and suggested she seek help adopting a healthy diet. Based on her bloodwork, we determined that some key lifestyle changes could probably help her achieve a prescription-free healthy lifestyle. Unfortunately, her insurance plan would not cover any of the appointments, education, or supplements she needed. In other words, they'd spend thousands of dollars a year as long as she stayed in the system and on the drugs. To break free, it would be out-of-pocket cost. She decided to go for it and hired me. Eight months later, she's almost 100% prescription free, lost a lot of weight, and has more energy.

Bottom line: **If there's a lab, procedure, test, or alternative medicine plan that would help you that is not covered within "the system", a hospital or a clinic may not even be able to offer or suggest it.**

At that point, it's up to you to find and purchase it on your own.

The good news is the effort is worth it.

You Have More Control Than You Think

Being in the driver's seat for your own health means making some changes that will help your body to heal itself instead of relying on prescriptions for disease management. The more information you have to make those changes, the better off you'll be—and that's what this book is about.

One important note: This book is only covering the basics at the surface. Each person reading this has a very specific individualized biochemistry. I cannot put my twenty-five-plus years of experience and seventeen-plus years of education into a small book. There is no one-size-fits-all approach to individual healing. Therefore, please allow this book to be your first step in your own journey, but it can't be a replacement for proper medical care by a licensed practitioner. It's meant to show you what's possible and how you can get there with direct guidance and help from a good Functional Medicine practitioner.

You can achieve true health. All you need is a guide in your journey to whole-body healing.

7 Reasons Why You Should Get Started Now

✓ **Thrive, don't just survive.**

Struggling to keep your head above water is exhausting and miserable. To be dependent on medications—sometimes lots of them—is not thriving; it is just a coping tool to keep pushing forward while never being 100 percent healed at any time. You were made to live an abundant life, fully present and in-the-moment, without co-dependency on medications.

✓ **More energy, less fatigue or pain.**

When the body's systems have been knocked out of balance, it's no wonder you have no energy left or have pain! Your mighty mitochondria powerhouses, found in each of your cells, just need some nutrient and mineral help for an initial boost! Your "fight-or-flight" system could be leaving you exhausted due to too much stress. Rather than just coping with more depleting habits and foods, you need the keys to help you get back on track.

✓ **One body, one chance, one here-and-now.**

Your lifestyle may be part of the reason you're suffering but making positive changes might be easier than you think. And isn't it worth at least considering? Think about it: We are only blessed with one body. We can honor it with nourishment, boundaries, resetting, and rest, or we can live a lifestyle that will keep us constantly out of balance. We all have a choice. Some may want to slowly make changes, and some desire or need to do so immediately due to major health issues. But it's important to make the changes—for yourself and no one else.

✓ Prevention is much cheaper than long-term medical bills.

As the Dalai Lama once said, we spend our lives losing our health to gain wealth, only to find ourselves losing our wealth in attempts to regain back our health. Self-care is as essential as the air you breathe. And small daily choices do *not* require expensive grocery bills. I can even show you how to eat healthily on a tight budget. If you add up costs on doctors, prescriptions, and chronic care over time and then compare that to the cost of preventative methods, you might be surprised at the difference.

✓ One pill leads to another...and who likes taking pills, anyway?

America's love affair with prescription meds is doing more harm than good. We now take more pills than ever. Just a few years ago, almost 1.3 million people in the US needed emergency hospital care due to adverse drug effects, and about 124,000 died from those events.[1] Unfortunately, if you're seeing multiple doctors or going to different pharmacies, these professionals may not be aware of which drugs you are taking, and therefore won't be able to consider potential interactions. And it's very easy to become non-functional with pain, rashes, diarrhea, anxiety, and sleep issues from the adverse effects of several drugs.

---

1   Teresa Carr, "Too Many Meds? America's Love Affair with Prescription Medication," *Consumer Reports*, August 3, 2017, https://www.consumerreports.org/prescription-drugs/too-many-meds-americas-love-affair-with-prescription-medication/.

✓ **Wake up rested—better sleep and mood.**

The cheapest step—and the first step—in regaining your health is to get more sleep. However, while I can tell you all of sleep's amazing health benefits, if you don't have the tools to help get you more of it, then the facts will do you no good. You probably are aware that environmental stress can affect your sleep, but did you know that things like your hormone levels can also be a factor? Better sleep equals less stress, a better mood, more energy, and more emotional and body awareness—all of which add up to a better life in general.

✓ **Feel confident in your own skin—and lose unwanted weight.**

I love seeing that glow on a client who has transformed into a different person. The hopeless, stressed-out, inflamed, out-of-balance, overweight, exhausted person who came to me in search of answers NOW walks in with bursting hope and a pep in their step, and feels alive again with the health they had longed to regain. That glow says it all! And you can have it. There IS hope. That's as good a reason as any to start now, isn't it?

Let's turn your symptoms into solutions.

CHAPTER 3

Take Control of Your Health

Hidden Lifestyle Costs of Being Unhealthy

Have you ever really sat down and thought about the impact your health has on every facet of your life? Do any of these apply to you?

- You miss important events (weddings, baby showers, birthday parties, etc.) due to your health problems.

- You can't perform as well at work, or you aren't able to work as much or at all.

- You can't perform tasks that should be routine—carrying in the groceries, going shopping in the first place, driving, etc.

- You can't join in or enjoy daily activities with others. Even something like playing a board game exhausts you.

- You can't process information because your condition or current medication puts you in a mental and emotional fog.

- Others who don't understand your suffering perceive you as unenthusiastic or lacking the desire to change.

- You feel hopeless and depressed.

- You lose touch with friends and family due to your inability to engage in those relationships as much.

- Your medical expenses prevent you from taking nice vacations or purchasing items you would really like to have.

You probably don't want to be in this situation, or you wouldn't be reading this book. So first off, let's figure out how you got here.

Your Health: Questionnaire

Can you think of a stressful time or event in your life that may have changed your health?

_____

_____

_____

_____

_____

_____

"I had been taking care of my parents while going through a divorce that I did not want. When my boss came in and told me I was getting laid off due to company financial issues, it was the straw that broke the camel's back for me. I had never had panic attacks before, and it scared me to death. I thought I was having a heart attack and went to the ER. I never thought about how all these events affected me. And now that I reflect back, I started having sleep and stomach issues right around when I went to the ER." —*John C. (Fayetteville, Arkansas)*

Compared to when you were truly healthy, how does your current condition affect your abilities and lifestyle?

_____

_____

_____

_____

How is your current condition affecting your relationships with your significant other, your family, or your friends?

_____

_____

_____

"I was a runner. It was my stress reliever and I really enjoyed it. Life just got busy, and I got more stressed. I was exhausted all the time and had no motivation to do anything because it would take me days to recover from it. I remember one day that my kids wanted me to climb Pinnacle Mountain with them, like I had done many times before. Immediately, I was overcome with fear just thinking about how many days it was going to set me back just to recover. This was my breaking point. I cried for days because my condition would not allow me to live my life." —Claire V. (Little Rock, Arkansas)

How is your current condition affecting your job/career or other financial income opportunities?

_____

_____

_____

What is your estimated annual financial burden each year for disease treatment (doctor visits, prescriptions, time off work without pay)?

_____

_____

_____

_____

_____

How is your health affecting your thoughts, beliefs, fears, or attitude?

_____

_____

_____

What does having energy and feeling well again mean to you?

_____

_____

_____

_____

"To be honest, I think I was depressed. I would cry over anything. Then I would beat myself up thinking I was being stupid about it. I just wasn't feeling normal—I was in a dark place. Then add the belly issues on to it. I would bloat after every meal, even small meals, and always felt like I needed coffee after meals just to get some energy. My son called the bloating a 'food baby.' I never realized that my gut health influenced my serotonin levels that much and had no idea I had food intolerance issues that gave me that food baby. You've also made me more aware of how food influences my body's reactions and energy." —_Stephanie (Searcy, Arkansas)_

What are your top three goals related to your health?

1. _____

2. _____

3. _____

Have you ever calculated the current financial costs of your medical bills, including doctor visits and medications? You might not realize how quickly it adds up. Try it now: for the previous year, list your estimated costs:

Medications (for the entire year, including over-the-counter ones):

_____

_____

_____

_____

Treatments:

_____

_____

Equipment and supplies you've had to buy:

_____

_____

_____

Other related costs such as unpaid time off work, lost hours due to sitting in the doctor's waiting room:

_____

_____

Total all those costs up:

_____

Now, add that amount to the additional cost of not being 100 percent present with family, work, and friends due to your compromised health (i.e., fatigue, depression, anxiety, panic attacks, hormone issues, etc.).

Is it worth your time and financial burden?

_____

IF you could get off medications and reclaim your health back, would you?

_____

What are the top three reasons you feel you won't be able to achieve better health? Be honest with yourself. What's really holding you back? What feels impossible? What makes you lose hope?

_____

_____

_____

_____

Did You Know? According to StatReports, Americans are being prescribed too many drugs, with 42 percent of adults over the age of sixty-five taking five or more medications daily. This creates a potentially dangerous situation for many. StatReports estimated that in 2018, one in five older Americans (ten million people) experienced an "adverse drug event."[2] The pharmaceutical industry's role in driving unnecessary and harmful medication use contributes to the over-prescription problem.

---

2   Shannon Brownlee and Judith Garber, "Overprescribed: High Cost Isn't America's Only Drug Problem," *STAT*, April 2, 2019, https://www.statnews.com/2019/04/02/overprescribed-americas-other-drug-problem/.

It Doesn't Have to Be This Way: Taking Charge of Your Health

Taking control of your health isn't a quick fix. And it doesn't put all the responsibility on someone else. A Functional Medicine approach asks you to work hand-in-hand with your practitioner to find the best solutions for your unique situation. To achieve better health, you need a few things:

- **Patience:** Wanting a "quick fix" causes a lot of obstacles. Be willing to accept that your changes will be long-term, and they will take time. Think "slow cooker" instead of "instant pot."

- **Knowledge:** Knowing the facts vs. the myths will help you make much better decisions.

- **Willingness to change:** Once you think about the cost of not changing vs. the cost of changing, getting into a new mindset might be easier than expected.

How Much Does It Cost to Do Small Daily Changes?

Remember: Your health isn't just physical. Your mind, body, and spirit all work together to heal you. Little things matter. With that in mind, here are some examples of small things I have patients do to start improving their health.

These do not take much time, but they can make a big difference over time—even if you can only do some of them.

MIND: Decrease Stress/
Perception of Stress, Increase Stress Resiliency

1. Meditate.

2. Practice yoga (or trauma yoga).

3. Do deep diaphragmatic breathing.

4. Take Epsom salts baths with lavender.

5. Sleep.

6. Practice mindfulness.

7. Improve internal dialogue.

8. See a trauma or stress coach or a mental health therapist.

BODY: *Feed Your Health—Literally!*

1. Eat healthier foods to reduce inflammation, thus reducing oxidative stress.

2. Cut out the sugar and processed foods. (I'll offer several nutrition-related tips in later chapters.)

3. Replenish your phytonutrients, vitamins, minerals, and probiotic strains through high-quality supplements.

4. Move more—increase your exercise and heart rate.

5. Adopt new daily healthy behavioral habits such as intuitive eating instead of emotional eating—take it one day at a time.

6. Improve your sleep to repair the body at the cellular level.

7. Practice deep diaphragmatic breathing several times daily.

8. Do grounding or earthing exercises and expose yourself to the sun at least fifteen minutes a day with no sunscreen chemicals.

SPIRIT: *Improve Your Mood, Mojo, Inner Peace, and Your "Vibes"*

"Spirit" is not necessarily about *religion*. It's about connection with others and with a Higher Power or a "bigger picture." It's about your belief system, relationships, and self-love.

1. Know that some things you do for the mind and body also affect spirit—especially things like meditations, guided imagery of healing, yoga, and earthing/grounding.

2. Find self-love and self-compassion by changing your internal dialogue from negative to positive thoughts.

3. Spend time with people you love and who lift you up, enriching relationships. Build your personal community.

4. Do something that feeds your creativity.

5. Spend time in nature, away from chaos, technology, toxicity, and pressures. Make "space" for yourself.

6. Let go of societal pressures, self-judgment, self-comparisons, and competition with others. Learn to just "be" and be happy in your own skin.

7. Laugh daily. It assists in producing the "feel-good hormones."

8. Find a connection to your personal understanding of a Higher Power. (I call Him "Pappa"; you might call yours God or not even use a specific name but just describe it as a sense of something greater than yourself.)

9. Consider Christian reiki.

Your energy level plays a role in how you feel about yourself, your day, and your overall attitude. We cannot separate what ails the body from what troubles the spirit.

8 Myths We Need to Bust

If you haven't been able to achieve your vision for good health, you could be falling for mistaken beliefs that keep you from even having hope—and if you have no hope, what's the use in trying?

Not sure what I'm talking about? See whether any of the below ring a bell:

1. **"My parents are obese, so I'm always going to be obese."**

    You are genetically predisposed to what your parents' DNA gave you. BUT knowing what is in your family genes gives you that cutting-edge knowledge of what TO do and what NOT TO do in lifestyle choices. If your parents are obese, then eating healthily, staying active, and getting proper sleep would be a MUST for you.

2. **"My lab ranges are 'normal,' so I must be okay."**

I know I've already mentioned this, so I hope you're still not falling for it. For some, a thyroid that tests like it's operating in the low-or high-"normal" range might not be giving them any symptoms, but another person with the same test results might have hair falling out, cold intolerance, early wakening issues, and more. So, it's imperative that we look at the symptoms instead of just looking at the lab ranges. It's important that you are HEARD, and your biochemistry is addressed.

3. **"It's normal to be on prescription drugs for the rest of my life."**

Do we need to go back and address the adverse effects of prescription drugs again? Or even the expense of them? Don't get me wrong; I'm not opposed to prescription meds. I've had to take quite a few in my lifetime. But there's a time and place for prescription medicines, and a pill is NOT always the answer for everything. Not all the time, but most of the time, poor lifestyle choices and unaddressed trauma or stress are what eventually lead to a body system's breakdown, resulting in the issues that conventional medicine treats with prescription drugs. So, if you can reverse or improve the lifestyle choices themselves (root causes) to get off the expensive prescription meds that cause adverse effects, would you?

4. **"I just need to eat less to lose weight (even though I am already eating only twelve hundred calories a day)."**

"Calories in" vs. "calories out" does not always work, especially when hormones are in the driver's seat. It's imperative we look at your nourishment and get rid of inflammation, heal the gut, reset or balance hormones, and get you plenty of water and sleep for weight loss to occur. Nurture the Mind-Body-Spirit.

5. **"It's expensive to eat healthily."**

We have gotten so accustomed to convenience. Fast food, processed foods, and highly preserved foods are destroying our health.

The SAD diet (Standard American Diet) does not improve or build up our health. So, when I hear "I don't like salads" or "eating healthy is too expensive and too time-consuming," what I'm really hearing is that you don't know HOW to eat healthily on a budget, you think that eating healthy means "salads only" (boring!), you don't understand the value of real food nourishment, and possibly you have not been taught how to cook or to choose food wisely. Real food is not rocket science, and you don't have to be a chef in order to bake, roast, or grill some vegetables and a piece of chicken or salmon.

6. **"It's too time-consuming to eat healthily."**

Preparing a meal shouldn't take more than thirty to forty-five minutes. My personal goal is a max of twenty-five minutes. And if I set aside one or maybe two days a week to chop fresh vegetables to make it easier for a quick meal through the week, then it saves even more time, PLUS I can buy in bulk for the week to save me money also. Saving time and money plus good health—isn't that what everyone wants anyway?

7. **"Several major health issues run in my family, so I will have them, too."**

As with obesity, the fact that a disease or ailment (such as diabetes or heart disease) runs in your family, that doesn't mean you will have it. I repeat: it does NOT mean you will have it. BUT, if you don't treat your body properly, then yes, you are much more likely to repeat your family history, and that means you need to be more aware of how to prevent that. Take a look at the Functional Medicine Tree illustration in the next chapter, which explains all of this in more detail.

8. **"I don't need mental health therapy; I have dealt with the stress of the death/sexual abuse/other traumatic experience on my own."**

Neurobiologist Robert Sapolsky wrote a book called *Zebras Don't Get Ulcers*, which explains the importance of allowing chronic stress and trauma to be "shaken off." Otherwise, it leads to an increased risk of disease and disability. Shaking it off—or grieving and addressing it—allows the nervous system to re-calibrate. Suppression, or just pretending it doesn't matter or trying to force it to go away, is like putting yourself in an emotional strait-jacket. It only increases post-traumatic stress disorder (PTSD), which results in chronic emotional, physical, and mental distress, contributing to high blood pressure, anxiety, depression, and addiction. Mental health therapists are trained in this area of healing.

Take Heart from Others' Success

Feeling even a glimmer of hope now? Maybe it will help you to hear from others who've thought their situation was hopeless but ended up being proven wrong.

Case Study #4: "Donald": Unaddressed Trauma from Son's Death

Donald's sister referred him to me after his health started suffering. He was an elder at his church, worked a full-time job, and had stuffed away his feelings after the tragic death of his son eight years before, never seeking therapy nor allowing himself to grieve. His doctor wanted to put him on anti-depressants and blood pressure medicine, both of which he refused. He had developed some gastrointestinal (GI) issues, as well as fatigue, depression, and insomnia.

Diagnosis: Suppressed and frozen emotions, which had led to further health issues of the heart, GI tract, and adrenal glands. Had a stressful position in his church while dealing with his own emotional, spiritual, and physical stress.

Goals:
- Address stored trauma both mentally and physically
- Improve the health of the nervous system and adrenals
- Decrease blood pressure

- Improve GI issues

- Improve mood

Treatment:
- Collaborated with a mental health therapist and trauma yoga therapist

- Diaphragmatic breathing four times daily

- Supplements to support the nervous system and adrenals

- Supplements and diet to improve blood pressure and GI issues

- Temporary supplements to increase serotonin production since he was not on an anti-depressant

Three months later: Donald had believed his health issues were ONLY based in his body. He didn't realize that his mind and spirit played a strong contributing role. "I bet you don't get men crying in your office much, do you?" he asked. "I apologize for that. You just don't know how much you have helped me. I'm glad my sister twisted my arm to come see you. Even though I thought I understood mind, body, spirit health, I now realize the Lord used you to redefine 'whole-body' healing. God was at work. I am starting to 'feel alive' again."

Case Study #5: "Amanda":
Mom Frustrated with Her Daughter's Care

Amanda came to me desperate and exhausted. She had been taking her daughter, now nineteen, to specialists since her daughter was thirteen. Her daughter had facial hair growth, irregular and heavy periods, weight gain that had affected her self-esteem, and migraines several times a month. She had been put on birth control at the age of thirteen to regulate her periods, but Amanda said it only made her gain more weight. Her daughter was also told to follow an eleven-hundred-calorie diet for weight loss. Amanda was a single mom, and her daughter's father was never involved in the girl's life. The weight gain Amanda's daughter experienced brought about undesirable attention from peers at school, increasing her stress and other issues. Because the girl had been suffering spiritually and emotionally from the weight gain, poor treatment by peers, low self-esteem and lack of her father's attention, and extreme low-calorie dieting, we performed several advanced tests to determine what hormonal and stress factors were at work.

Diagnosis: Amanda's daughter experienced all areas of imbalance in mind, body, spirit. Testing confirmed estrogen dominance, PCOS issues, cortisol imbalance, and neurotransmitter imbalance. Most likely, her migraines were brought on partly from hormone imbalance but mostly from dehydration and insufficient magnesium, which could be depleted by stress (we'll get to that in later chapters).

Goals:
- Complete whole-body healing

- Get PCOS under control without the use of birth control

- Weight loss to improve self-esteem

- Stop the migraines

Treatment:
- Two types of inositol with diindolylmethane (DIM) for PCOS

- A diabetic-type meal plan (more than thirteen-hundred calories) for controlling insulin

- Adaptogen support for adrenals

- Supplements to decrease migraines

- Diaphragmatic breathing and yoga

- Three hours of dancing to her favorite music each week

- Encouragement for Amanda's daughter to see a mental health therapist due to absent father and trauma from being made fun of at school

Three Months Later: Amanda's daughter had lost forty-three pounds and walked with confidence. She'd had only one migraine in three months, and her last period was only three days late instead of twenty. "She decided the day she left your office she was no longer taking the birth control," Amanda told me. "She saw her friend's mental health therapist several times and was motivated to stick with the treatment plan when her facial hair started going away. This has been life-changing for her. I truly believe she's almost 'whole-body' healed. I can't thank you enough for all your help!"

Ready to Learn More?

Now, for more of that "knowledge" part. Are you ready to learn more about how you can help your body heal itself? Let's take a look in the next chapter.

CHAPTER 4

How Functional Medicine Works

Getting to Root Causes

From the age of five, I grew up pulling weeds for hours a day in our family garden, up until the day I left for college. If I only pulled out what was above the surface, I got in trouble. When I was younger, I never understood WHY we could not just let those weeds grow. In my little mind, I thought it was a complete waste of my summertime. Pulling those weeds around our plants didn't matter...the plant was still going to give us the vegetable or fruit. And if I only pulled the weed top that was on the surface, that should be enough to satisfy my parents. I mean, it made the garden look pretty, and that should be sufficient, right?

Hmmm...

Fast forward thirty-plus years. While out watering my garden early one morning with Kari Jobe music playing from the phone in my pocket, I reached down to pull up a weed, making sure I pulled up the root. What did this adult know now that the kid before hadn't?

My parents' gardening lessons so long ago had (eventually) taught me something very important.

If I only pulled off what could be seen above the surface, the weed's root would continue to grow deep underground, affecting my garden plants' root systems too.

It could also possibly spread and choke out/kill off my vegetation. Plus, the weeds would pull nutrients away from my garden plants. This would deprive the garden of the full nutrition the plants needed to produce our vegetables and fruits—possibly reducing our harvest.

So, while taking care of only the surface might look pretty on the outside, the issues are still there, deep underneath.

I also know now that I need to pay close attention not just to what I'm taking out of my garden and how but also what I'm putting IN. What's adding (or not) to the soil quality around my plant's roots? Whatever is in that soil will be in my fruit and vegetables—and eventually in me. The quality of the soil affects the harvest, too.

So, what's my point?
Our environment is like soil quality. It should nourish our "plant" (our person), providing mental and spiritual growth and nutrient-dense foods for our body. Our environment plays a major role in feeding our health and improving the quality of the fruit/vegetables produced (healthy quality of life, strong potential, and absence of disease).

The weeds (the things in a person's environment that suffocate him or her and dry up the spirit) need to be pulled up at the root and extracted. These include things like stress/trauma, inflammation, and/or toxins, all of which choke out the body's health and ability to fight disease, as well as the mental and emotional capability to recover from stress. Addressing only the symptoms with drugs while leaving the "root causes" behind will allow these "weeds" to continue suffocating the Mind-Body-Spirit growth. That will prevent the person from harvesting a full "crop" of health and healthy life experiences. This progressive erosion of the personal "garden" will continue until the true issues are addressed—which could potentially mean an entire lifetime of suffering if they are not.

Functional Medicine Can Help

Functional Medicine dives deep into the root cause of disease, looking into the history and current state of all aspects of Mind-Body-Spirit. Functional Medicine practitioners are like health detectives. The clues we investigate are bodily symptoms, trauma history, lifestyle patterns, eating patterns, food choices, movement, sleep, stress, relationships, etc. With these, we formulate a timeline showing when health started to go awry. From there, we formulate a plan from the ground up for healing. We know that sickness is an accumulative thing. It does not show up overnight. For true, lasting healing, we need to dig deep into the "root," addressing the when and how it started.

The goal? To wean patients off prescription med dependency, heal and restore the body, and create a whole-body healing that helps people get their energy and lives back.

When looking at the root, we ask if the person is getting the right nourishment of:

- Sleep/Relaxation

- Exercise/Movement

- Nutrition/Water

- Relationships/Networks/Spiritual/Social

- Healthy Microorganisms

And we also look to see if anything is decreasing the quality of nourishment of the Mind-Body-Spirit. Stress burdens, trauma, environmental pollutants, or unhealthy microorganisms can block the healing process.

The common conventional approach is to ask, "What drug matches up with this disease?" But Functional Medicine asks, "What is creating these symptoms in the first place?" or "What is the upstream (mental, emotional, physical) issue that has created this downstream symptom?" Getting those answers requires us to look into the person's biochemistry from all angles to learn what affected the Mind-Body-Spirit.

Nutrition is the foundation for body health. With my two-and-a-half decades of experience as a registered dietitian, along with my

Functional-Medicine-trained detective skills, I can look at my patients' health issues from even greater depth.

Mind-Body-Spirit—All Affect Each Other

Might I step out of my role as a Functional Medicine dietitian and just be your gut-honest friend for a moment? I just need to lay a very touchy subject out on the table here, or I would never be able to forgive myself. If you have endured trauma, PTSD, or grief, it's imperative that your body heals from it—which means that your mind must heal from it.

Mental health therapists specialize in helping people heal in those areas where the brain's thought processes and emotions are affected. I'm not that person, but I will collaborate with that person to help you. What I am is your body-healing person, and hopefully, I'm a portion of your spirit-healing as well. That means I need to be your biggest supporter in seeing a mind-healing person. They actually help me to help YOU fully heal, which is my ultimate goal.

Remember before, when I touched on the fact that your mind, body, and spirit all work together to keep you healthy? That sometimes means that multiple practitioners need to collaborate to help you. And that's a good thing.

Did you know that EVERY cell in your body—including the nervous system—has memory?[3] When a person's spirit is still affected by past traumatic experiences, it often goes unnoticed until a symptom manifests in the mind (depression, panic attacks, anxiety, etc.)

The body keeps the score, and eventually, it will speak.

I want you to understand that your Mind-Body-Spirit connection is inseparable. It is an integrated triad...a triune. Some spiritual belief systems recognize this tightly interwoven triune also. Whatever you believe, it's just important to understand that when one of these facets is affected, the other two are affected. Mental effects will present themselves in a

---

3   "Memory—New Research Reveals Cells Have It Too," Evolution
    News, November 19, 2018, https://evolutionnews.org/2018/11/
    memory-new-research-reveals-cells-have-it-too/.

host of physical and emotional anxiety-induced illnesses or simply erode your physical health. I learned this the hard way while living through it on my own healing journey.

Functional Medicine practitioners look at a person's timeline from pre-birth up until the present. Something may have affected the Mind-Body-Spirit at a younger age, though it wasn't noticed. If not addressed, it will create a chain reaction, causing another symptom that affects another aspect of the Mind-Body-Spirit. This, in turn, will create yet another symptom...and it goes on. Compounded symptoms/effects over a period of time will eventually surface to the point that the effects show up in lab work. They also show up in how you handle stress. They can eventually manifest as larger issues, such as some form of Adrenal Dysfunction, leaky gut, anxiety, panic attacks, chronic fatigue, low libido or heavy periods, and poor sleep patterns, to name a small few.

If you are taking a prescription drug to address symptoms, you can:

1. Continue the drug without addressing the root cause. Unfortunately, you will likely eventually end up on other drugs to treat the first drug's side effects.

2. Continue the drug WHILE addressing the root cause—with the goal of healing and eventually weaning you off the drug.

3. Stop the drug and seek root-cause healing with both temporary and permanent lifestyle changes. These include things like targeted food choices, natural vitamins, minerals, adaptogens, aminos, phytonutrients, mental health therapy, etc.

A Functional Medicine approach uses Nos. 2 and 3, depending on the individual's condition and health. But there is definitely a need for the standard model of care shown in No. 1, especially in cases of acute conditions, infection, physical trauma, and emergencies. For those situations, I'm beyond grateful for that resource!

The field of Functional Medicine, with its holistic approach to healing the whole person (Mind-Body-Spirit), is finding solutions to many chronic conditions such as digestive issues, allergies, metabolic issues, neurological issues, and hormonal imbalances—all of which cause many Americans to suffer daily.

WHY we address the triad of Mind-Body-Spirit:

We are created in a way that each aspect affects the other two. We can NOT separate the three when it comes to whole-body healing.

Example:

Human beings develop PTSD because of frozen emotions. In cases of childhood abuse, the child cannot escape and has to freeze his/her emotions **(mind)*** because the parent is often the source of the trauma.

Suppression of PTSD over a long time causes excess energy to be trapped in our **bodies** (I call this "living in a straitjacket"). This creates tension and mental distress (all of which affect the **spirit**).

Continual activation of the stress response can lead to **body** ailments such as high blood pressure, clogged arteries, and brain changes leading to anxiety, depression, addiction, HPA-Axis Adrenal Dysfunction, low libido, and low functioning thyroid, to name a few.

*Veronique Mead, "ME/CFS and Freeze: A Metabolic State of Hibernation that Is Not in Your Head," Chronic Illness Trauma Studies, September 14, 2018, https://chronicill-nesstraumastudies.com/mecfs-freeze/

Who Practices Functional Medicine?

Functional Medicine Practitioners are those already in the medical field, typically for several years, that decided to further their education:

- Medical Doctors or Doctors of Osteopathic Medicine

- Physician Assistants

- Registered Dietitians

- Nurse Practitioners

- Chiropractors

- Naturopathic Doctors

- Pharmacists

The Functional Medicine Tree Perspective

Here's another analogy. Think of your body's systems like a large tree. The roots represent the foundation of your tree, where the nourishment starts. The nourishment (good or bad) that you're feeding your roots will start to eventually affect the tree's health all the way up to the top branch and through every leaf, nut, or fruit it might produce.

The health of the visible parts of your tree (trunk, branches, leaves, nuts, and fruit) results from the health of the invisible parts under the surface—each tree root. Your tree roots need proper sleep and relaxation, exercise and movement, nutrition and hydration, stress resiliency (from daily stressors, trauma, and environmental stress such as pollution, mold, and toxins), and good relationships.

The trunk of your big tree represents your genetic predisposition, outside influences, and life experiences.

What you feed your tree roots will determine what kind of tree branch you will grow. Tree branches could be full of heart disease, diabetes, obesity, HPA-Axis Adrenal Dysfunction, thyroid dysfunction, sex hormone dysfunction, etc. OR a tree branch could be completely healthy and void of dysfunction.

Though you can't see the roots of your large tree, the health of what we do see above ground will reveal how you nourish them. So, by nourishing the roots, healing the roots, tending to the roots, you get a healthier tree in spite of genetic predisposition.

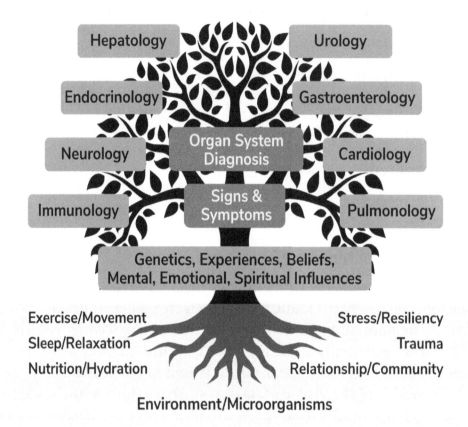

Alternative Healing as Complement, Not Competitor

Ancient Eastern medicine has been around much longer than Western/conventional medicine and incorporates fewer prescription pharmaceuticals and more holistic approaches to healing. Obviously, we need to be discerning and should not fall for any "woo-woo medicine" or "snake oil" that comes along. But many evidence-based scientific studies prove other modes of healing are worthy of looking into. These include acupuncture, chiropractic medicine, meridian therapy, massage therapy, holistic medicine, homeopathy, Christian reiki, trauma yoga, mental health therapy, and of course, Functional Medicine, to name a few.

It's not unusual for me to prescribe complementary therapies like the above in addition to what I am doing for a patient. Far from being competing therapies, they actually work along with the Functional Medicine approach and help address the full set of needs related to the patient's mind, body, and spirit.

CHAPTER 5

A Major Health Culprit: Stress

Are You "Running from a Bear"?

One way to look at how your mind, body, and spirit all affect each other is to look at the effects of stress.

Suppose you are walking along in the woods, and suddenly, you run across a bear. Your body instantly goes into **Acute Stress Response** called **"Fight-or-Flight" Mode.** This physiological reaction occurs when you perceive or experience a harmful event, attack, or threat to your survival (real or imagined). The fear that activates this response can be perceived or real. The hypothalamus in the brain activates the **sympathetic nervous system** by sending signals to the **adrenal glands.** The adrenal glands produce a secretion of catecholamine, norepinephrine, and epinephrine (also known as adrenaline). As the adrenaline circulates through the body, it brings on a number of physiological changes; for example, the heart beats faster, and blood pressure goes up. Adrenaline also triggers the release of blood sugar (glucose) and fats from storage sites in the body. These flood the bloodstream for the urgent supply of energy that can allow you to run from the bear. You can handle this Acute Stress Response every so often. **The problem is when you experience it daily or even multiple times in the day...**like you are constantly running from not only one bear but many. **This leads to Chronic Stress Mode**, or running from multiple bears all the time, which soon will keep your adrenals pumping out the stress hormone cortisol when it should be at rest.

Cortisol, your stress hormone, gives you life. It should be high in the morning for energy and low at night so that your sleep hormone melatonin can kick in. When cortisol remains elevated because you are spending too much time in fight-or-flight mode, the more fatigue and brain fog you will have, increasing your risk of constipation, inflammation, improper toxin removal, and poor sleep.

These symptoms create further issues, adding further stress (yet another bear!) internally for your body's internal systems to work properly. Plus, other hormones start to become greatly affected by this, due to a chain reaction. Such hormones are estrogen, testosterone, progesterone, as well as neurotransmitter dopamine (for focus, mood, motivation) and serotonin (your natural anti-depressant).

When you add more and more bears as you run, you will never get into relaxation mode, the lack of which will conflict with parasympathetic and sympathetic nervous system balance and breathing.

A "bear" can signify any form of stress on the body:

- Disease (diabetes, poor heart health, poor gut health, inflammation, etc.)

- Poor diet (the SAD diet, sugar, highly processed food, etc.)

- Inadequate sleep

- Situational stress (financial/work-related/relationship, trauma, death of a loved one, etc.)

- Environmental factors (exposure to mold, toxins, chemicals, etc.)

Living in Chronic Stress Mode will overwhelm the chain reactions from your brain to your adrenal glands, which is also referred to as the Hypothalamus-Pituitary-Adrenal (HPA) Axis. This Chronic Stress Mode leads to "Adrenal Dysfunction" or "adrenal fatigue." The second term is a little misleading, so I will call it **Adrenal Dysfunction** from here on out. To learn more about it, see chapter 5.

Staying in Chronic Stress Mode will eventually take a toll on the health of the gut, thyroid, nervous system, adrenal hormones, and sex hormone production. It easily brings about anxiety, panic attacks, low libido, insomnia, or depression. This, in turn, affects your spirit, mental clarity, energy level, sleep, mood, attitude...and you become super-sensitive to stress due to loss of stress resiliency.

The Autonomic Nervous System

Let's break the nervous system I just described down into its two parts:

1. **Parasympathetic:** Your Rest and Digest Mode. It's like your toes are in the sand; you're relaxed and have not a care in the world. We all would love to stay here, but it's just not reality, right?

2. **Sympathetic:** You are RUNNING FROM A BEAR! Your mind doesn't shut down, your body is never at rest, you're wound tight, you have a history of trauma that hasn't been addressed, you stay in constant cortisol production and stressed out, you have no sleep or have trouble falling asleep, and your immune system is suffering. Staying here is Fight-or-Flight Mode.

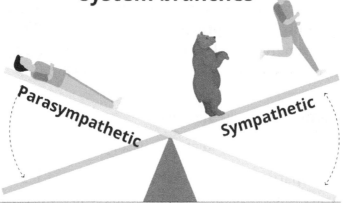

Homeostasis is a dynamic balance between the autonomic nervous system branches

Rest and Digest	Fight or Flight
Relaxed	Stressed/Cortisol release
Belly breathing	Shallow breathing
Slower heart rate	Increases heart rate & BP
Increases intestinal activity	Decreases intestinal activity
Relaxes & repairs muscles	Breaks down muscles
Less risk of weight gain	Weight gain

Here's the kicker...you need BOTH the sympathetic and parasympathetic systems but in BALANCE...in an ebb and flow, just like ocean waves coming in and rolling out, coming in and rolling out again.

It gives us resilience to stress and keeps the immune system strong.

Ones living in Chronic Stress Mode rarely feel the effects of the parasympathetic because their stressed-out bodies have a difficult time switching out of the sympathetic. This condition is called "Sympathetic Dominance."

Common Characteristics of People Living in Chronic Stress Mode and Sympathetic Dominance:[4]

- ✓ One's upbringing in an unhealthy environment—abusive or absent parenting; also, parents demanding perfection; certain "religions" instead of "relationship"

- ✓ People pleasers

- ✓ Workaholics

- ✓ Overachievers

- ✓ History of physical and/or sexual abuse

- ✓ Witnessing a tragic event

- ✓ Empaths

- ✓ Type A personalities

Living in Chronic Stress and Sympathetic Dominance

Stress can lead to many mental, emotional, and physical challenges, including:

- Digestive issues such as chronic bloating, stomach pain, diarrhea, constipation, not digesting food properly, etc.

- Feeling "wired" but tired, or "wound up" tight

- Low body temperature

- Experiencing anxiety or panic attacks (for people with anxiety disorders, the stress system never shuts down)[5]

---

4   Dr. Lawrence Wilson, "Sympathetic Dominance," LD Wilson Consultants, Inc., Accessed February 23, 2021, https://www.drlwilson.com/Articles/SYMPATHETIC%20DOMINANCE.htm.

5   Berit Brogaard, "How Deep Relaxation Affects Brain Chemistry," *Psychology Today*, March 31, 2015, https://www.psychologytoday.com/us/blog/the-mysteries-love/201503/how-deep-relaxation-affects-brain-chemistry.

- Unable to slow down mentally

- Feeling chronically rushed

- Feeling like you have to constantly be doing something

- Dilated pupils

- Insomnia

- Fast pulse

- Lowered immunity

- Increased blood pressure and blood sugar

- Increased sweating

- Tight shoulder and neck muscles

- Constant fatigue

- Fearful

- Anxious

- Nightmares

- Nail-biting

- Temporomandibular jaw disorder (TMJ)

- Tension headaches

How to Correct Sympathetic Dominance from Chronic Stress

Some people want an instant pot instead of a slow cooker. Unfortunately, with the nervous system, you have to take the slow cooker route. Instant changes won't happen rapidly. Persistence will make progress happen.

I have to remind my patients that they did not just get here overnight. But the following changes to daily habits will definitely get the system back into a balance much more quickly.

1. **Clean up your diet.** Most people in sympathetic dominance will be eating on the run, consuming processed and/or sugar-loaded, man-made foods. It's pretty common to over-consume caffeine as well. As the old saying goes, "You are what you eat." Eat colorful, nutrient-dense food that is REAL, not processed, which gives you lots of vitamins and minerals.

2. **Get enough sleep!** You need seven to nine hours of uninterrupted sleep. This allows the body's nervous system to relax and rejuvenate. Need help in this area? Try the suggestions on sleep in chapter 9.

3. **Take adaptogens,** such as ashwagandha, holy basil, and rhodiola, to help calm the adrenals, which also helps calm down the nervous system.

4. **Supplement with phosphatidylserine,** an amino acid that helps push down cortisol to help your melatonin kick in. Melatonin is your sleep hormone!

5. **Magnesium,** magnesium, magnesium! Unfortunately, our American soil is becoming depleted of this mineral. It will down-regulate the sympathetic nervous system, helping balance it with the parasympathetic.

6. **Meditate.** This was something that I ran from for a while. I had a stigma in my head that it was ONLY for Buddhists or monks. Pfft! I've learned a lot on this health journey! Evidence-based science proves that daily meditation helps to heal and reset your nervous system slowly.

7. **Take warm baths** with Epsom salts and lavender oil. Rarely does anyone want to turn this down! The body soaks up the magnesium in the Epsom salt, and the lavender essential oil is calming to the limbic system (in the brain), which calms the mind and can even induce sleep.

8. **Decrease high-intensity activity.** You remember me saying this was a huge mental challenge for me? But it's ever so true...just do yoga, trauma yoga, or casual walks instead.

9. **Say NO.** Know your boundaries and stick with them. Don't overload yourself. Make a list of top priorities and stick with it!

10. **Seek mental health therapy** if trauma has ever happened in your life.

11. **Laugh!** Take time out to RELAX and bring some FUN back into your life.

12. **Practice diaphragmatic breathing technique.** You can do this several times a day, and no one will know you are doing it!

13. **Listen to calming brainwave or bilateral music.** There are a ton of options on YouTube.

14. **Try red light therapy to increase melatonin.**

CHAPTER 6

HPA Axis, Adrenal Dysfunction, and Issues

Are You an Overwhelmed Baker?

Along the same lines with "running from bears" that I described in the previous chapter, suppose you love to bake, and so you decided to run your own bakery. However, you keep getting more and more orders, and you eventually can't keep up doing what you used to love to do. This is exactly what is happening to your HPA axis and adrenal gland when you become overwhelmed and lose the passion for things you normally feel excited about.

Being overwhelmed and exhausted will create inflammation within the body and flare up autoimmune system problems. So, pain, arthritis, and fatigue set in. It's a hamster wheel of stress.

Reaching for Quick Energy

Another problem is that when we're overwhelmed, we reach for things to give us more energy, such as coffee, caffeine, sugar, or energy drinks, but they will leave us even more exhausted, depleted, and overwhelmed.

A small cup of coffee in the morning is okay, but randomly drinking caffeine throughout the day brings about an irregular adrenal cortisol rhythm and creates issues with anxiety, further sleep disturbances, and weight gain from excess cortisol surges. Our blood pressure rises, and we are put on medications, then those medications create further nutrient deficiencies ....

The Endocrine Pyramid: Root Cause Healing from Ground Up

The endocrine system is complex, so I'll just bring out some main points to show what most of my clients face yet do not understand. **To keep it as simple as I can, I will not be able to mention many of the other facets.**

Imagine a pyramid of three layers. The foundation, which is the biggest, is the Adrenal Gland Hormones layer. The middle layer is Thyroid Hormones. And the top layer is Sex Hormones.

Endocrine Pyramid
Simplified

**Sex
Hormones**
Progesterone
Estrogen
Testosterone (*libido*)

Thyroid Hormones
TSH (technically a pituitary hormone)
Total T4, Free T4
Total T3, Free T3
Reverse T3

Adrenal Hormones
Cortisol (*stress hormone*) & Cortisone
Epinephrine & Norepinephrine
Testosterone & DHEA
Aldosterone (*regulates blood pressure*)

The Complexity of the Endocrine System

The endocrine system is a series of hormones that respond to the message of other hormones. Imagine it much like a domino effect. This involves several routes of hormone messaging/signaling:

1. Hypothalamus-Pituitary-Adrenal (HPA) Axis

2. Hypothalamus-Pituitary-Thyroid (HPT) Axis

3. Hypothalamus-Pituitary-Gut (HPG) Axis

Let's dive into a few areas of the endocrine system. Three of them, the adrenal glands, thyroid, and the GI tract, all start with the brain's hypothalamus and pituitary glands, where stress is interpreted or perceived. The stress put on the body will have the sex hormones (testes/ovaries) speaking to the brain and thyroid in a slightly different way than usual.

The Bottom Tier: Addressing the Foundation of the Pyramid

The foundation is crucial because everything else rests on it. It's holding everything up! You can't just address the top layers until you address the foundation, or you will ALWAYS be repairing, putting the "bandages" on the symptoms. The foundation HAS to be a solid, firm foundation.

Do you suffer from low libido? Your testosterone or DHEA might be low, and you could go on hormone replacement meds...but do you want to remain on them forever if your body can eventually produce them on its own?

And how about your hair thinning out? Aren't you tired of staying cold-natured and tired all the time? Your thyroid hormones might be a little in the hypothyroid range. Hormone replacement could help, but do you want to remain on hormone supplements all your life if you can address the problem simply by increasing a certain mineral or avoiding a certain food?

Taking all kinds of different hormone replacements will soon create a huge balancing game for your practitioner, and you are the one who suffers through it until it's figured out. Unfortunately, your body is ever-changing...which means the balancing game will never really end.

So How Do We Fix the Foundation AND Feel "Normal" Again?
We have to look to see what is affecting the adrenal gland. The typical question is, "What is making the HPA Axis overstimulated, which makes the adrenal glands shoot off too much or too little cortisol?"

Take a look at the following stressors that prompt cortisol production.

Which of these apply to you?

Life Issues

____ Financial Pressures   ____ Death of a Loved One

____ Marital Stress   ____ Unwanted Unemployment

____ Emotional Stress   ____ Psychological Stress

____ Fear   ____ Negative Attitudes & Beliefs

Body Issues

____ Allergies   ____ Prescription Drugs

____ Wound Healing   ____ Infections: Acute & Chronic

Lifestyle

____ Smoking   ____ Lack of OR Excessive Exercise

____ Over Exertion   ____ Lack of Relaxation

____ Toxins   ____ Poor Eating Habits

Diet:

____ Coffee (Two or More Cups/Day)   ____ Coffee in the Evenings for Energy

____ Caffeine   ____ Sugar

____ White Flour Products   ____ Lack of Good Quality Food

Total the above that pertain to you: _____

If you can relate to at least five of these, then you are either headed into Adrenal Dysfunction, or you are already IN Adrenal Dysfunction.

The above issues are all stressors. These stressors lead to new stressors because of the stress hormone called cortisol, which I've mentioned several times. Remember that bear?

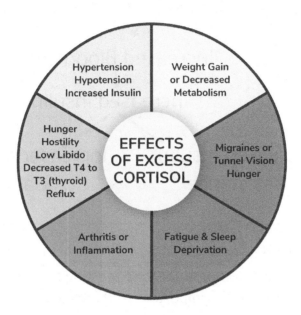

When a person remains in Chronic Stress Response, whether it be due to a perceived threat or a lack of resilience to stress due to continued stress over time, cortisol eventually takes a toll on the body in many areas, including the immune system, cardiovascular health, neurochemistry (depression, mood, anxiety), and it messes with the body's metabolism and blood sugar control (metabolic syndrome, which leads to diabetes).

Cortisol Effects on Blood Sugar: Weight Gain and Metabolic Syndrome

When cortisol rises from constant stress, the sugar cravings set in. WHY? Sugar stimulates another hormone called **serotonin, which is our calming and relaxing hormone.** And as cortisol increases, it will increase blood sugars in an effort to provide the body with energy to run from the bear. The rise of glucose and extra intake of sugar eventually lead to insulin resistance. This soon will bring on weight gain and Metabolic Syndrome...and suddenly, you learn you have diabetes, heart disease, mood disorders, and a poor immune system!

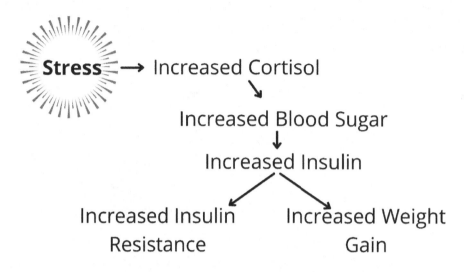

Did you know?

The quality of the foods you eat isn't the only thing to think about. Believe it or not, it's also important to think about the foods you're eating together!

I tell my patients—especially diabetics—that they should never eat a carb alone. NEVER. A carb needs to be eaten (paired) with at least one protein and/or protein-fat "buddy." That even goes for healthy carbohydrates, made by our Creator. Pairing carbohydrates will help balance your blood sugars, decreasing your sugar cravings and your risk of diabetes. That carb-craving roller coaster is no joke...so to prevent it, just pair that healthy carb with its buddy or buddies.

Middle Tier: The Thyroid

Let's go back to that Endocrine Pyramid. Cortisol is produced on the bottom layer, the foundation. As cortisol production increases, it begins to affect the thyroid.

Here's the route by which your thyroid hormones are produced:

Hypothalamus→Pituitary→Thyroid→T4→T3→into cells for energy

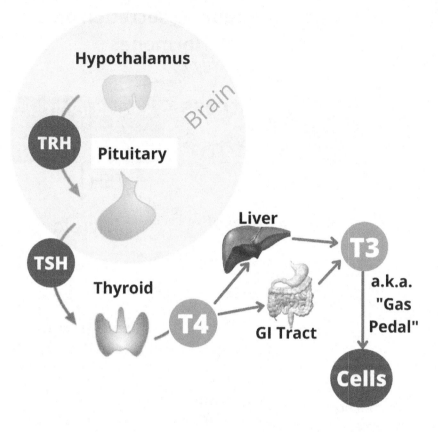

The hypothalamus and pituitary (in the brain) tell the thyroid (in the neck) how much T4 (hormone) to produce. T4 converts to T3 (the active thyroid hormone) in the liver and gut (if both are healthy). **T3 is our gas pedal to our body's energy**! We want the gas pedal on, not the brakes.

Problems with Thyroid and Elevated Cortisol

When the body is stressed (physical and or emotional), it secretes cortisol and inhibits the T4 from producing T3. So, you guessed it...it inhibits our gas pedal. It makes the body put on the brakes instead. The degree to which the brakes are being pushed is measured in a lab test for something called "Reverse T3 (rT3)." This test is rarely done as part of the thyroid panel. And most insurance companies will not pay for it; therefore, you will most likely have to pay out of pocket for it.

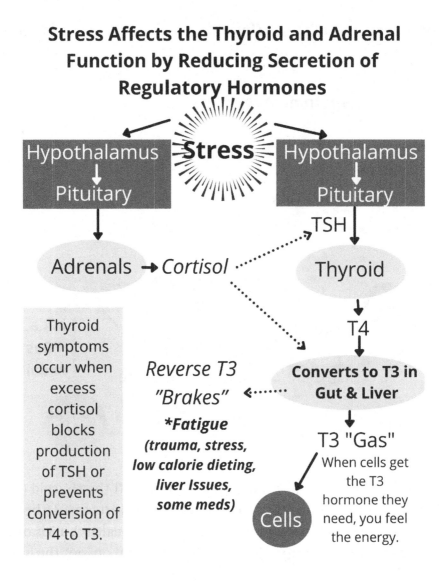

Reverse T3 is best thought of as an anti-thyroid metabolite, meaning that it is something your body creates to slow down thyroid function... it's the brake pedal. With it present, you will feel fatigued and symptoms of hypothyroidism, even if your T3 lab levels are "normal" because rT3 is blocking T3's effects to protect the thyroid. So, if you have experienced any of the following, it is crucial you get an rT3 lab drawn with your other thyroid labs:

1. **Trauma, PTSD, Emotional and/or Physical Stress.** Long-term high stress can push cortisol high, pushing T4 to convert to the inactive Reverse T3, which causes hypothyroid symptoms. This is called Secondary Hypothyroidism, and it is correctable.

2. **Calorie Restriction.** Restricting calorie intake by large amounts to lose weight can have the opposite effect. It stresses the body and puts on the brakes quickly, which will actually make the thyroid sluggish...and a sluggish thyroid will bring about weight gain.

3. **Inflammation.** This causes a spike in rT3.[6] In my experience, most cases of inflammation are caused by eating low-quality foods daily. Sugary foods, processed foods, and foods made with industrial seed oils are often the culprit. Inflammation will also affect the gut health and absorption of nutrients, which I will discuss later.

4. **Nutrient Deficiencies.** Nutrients help certain enzymes function in your body. Your body may want to convert the T4 to T3 but is slow in doing so if you are too low on zinc[7], selenium, vitamin E, and vitamin A. Nutrient deficiencies can actually increase the conversion to rT3. Zinc and selenium tend to help more with T4 to T3 conversion, while vitamins A and E help more with thyroid cellular activity and sensitivity.

5. **Unhealthy Gut or Liver.** Conversion of T4 to T3 takes place in the liver and gut. If either is not healthy, then the conversion will not take place. Your gut is a huge source of hormones, immune function, thyroid conversion, and neurotransmitters.

---

6   Rainer H. Straub, "Interaction of the Endocrine System with Inflammation: A Function of Energy and Volume Regulation," *Arthritis Research and Therapy* 16, no.1 (February 2014): 203, https://dx.doi.org/10.1186/ar4484.

7   S. Nishiyama, Y Futagoishi-Suginohara, M. Matsukura, T. Nakamura, A. Higashi, M. Shinohara, and I. Matsuda, "Zinc Supplementation Alters Thyroid Hormone Metabolism in Disabled Patients with Zinc Deficiency," *Journal of the American College of Nutrition* 13, no.1(1994): 62-67, https://doi.org/10.1080/07315724.1994.10718373.

Any gut dysfunction can compromise these functions. At least 20 percent of your T4 to T3 conversion takes place here. An unhealthy gut will increase the rT3, so addressing all gut issues is paramount in addressing rT3 levels.

6. **Lack of Sleep.** You should be getting at least seven to nine hours of *quality, uninterrupted* sleep each night, or it creates high stress on the body.

I also use some great evidence-based healing supplements with my clients that help in supporting the thyroid's overall function. Of course, along with the supportive supplements, a healthy diet—gluten-free specifically—will help support thyroid health.

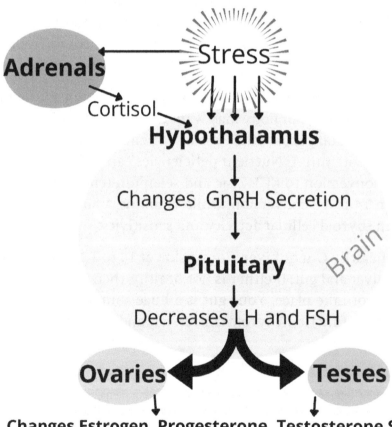

Changes Estrogen, Progesterone, Testosterone Synthesis
(Low Libido, Heavy or Irregular Periods, PCOS, Migraines, Brain Fog, Poor Quality Sleep)

Top Tier: Sex Hormone Production "Stress Steal"

Aside from the female needing connection in order for intimacy to occur, which assists in libido (this is part of the "**spirit**" in mind-body-spirit)—stress also plays a role.

When under stress (or "living in the straitjacket"), the body prioritizes "survival" as cortisol increases. As it increases in the brain (specifically the hypothalamus), the sex-regulating hormones start to decrease, thus decreasing the synthesis of the sex hormones.

This occurs because the hypothalamus secretes a hormone called Gonadotropin Reducing Hormone (GnRH) that in turn works with the pituitary to regulate the sex hormones in both men and women.

But if there is too much cortisol in the body, the hypothalamus does not produce as much GnRH, which then decreases the activities of the pituitary and, thus, at the end of the "stream," the sex hormones, too.

Some call this the "cortisol steal," which is a bit misleading since there are quite a few steps that take place between the stress and the outcome of low sex hormone production. I prefer to call it the "stress steal" instead. The "downstream" effects show up in various ways.

Low Libido? Blame it on the stress steal, decreasing your testosterone synthesis. (Or work on the connection/relationship with your significant other so that the "spirit" part of mind-body-spirit is addressed.)

Irregular monthly periods? Blame it on the stress steal, decreasing the GnRH synthesis.

Anxious or depressed? Insomnia? You guessed it ... it is commonly, but not always, the stress steal.

But before we just point fingers at the stress steal, we need to investigate further upstream to find out WHY you need more cortisol. What stressors are going on in your life that demand excessive cortisol production—for instance, a poor diet? Emotional stress? Poor-quality sleep? How can we treat those issues to prevent further damage?

In summary, the upstream effects of excessive stress lead to excessive cortisol production and decreased GnRH, creating downstream problematic health issues that can easily be treated by addressing the upstream issues instead of just using hormone replacement or birth control to "put a bandage on the symptoms." These are far easier Solutions to the Symptoms.

Because of high insulin levels (from cortisol or from poor diet), such as are common in PCOS, the ovaries won't receive the correct signals from the pituitary to produce the hormones it needs for the eggs to mature. Since no eggs mature or are released, ovulation does not occur and the hormone progesterone is not made, which stops or makes the menstrual cycle irregular, creates brain fog and poor-quality sleep.

So, Is Your Root Cause Diagnosis HPA-Axis Adrenal Dysfunction?

Remember the examples of running from a bear or being an overwhelmed baker? As your adrenals are constantly signaled to produce cortisol from chronic stress, the cortisol will create issues with the thyroid, the sex hormones, the gut, and insulin. This is the initial stage of Adrenal Dysfunction and HPA Axis issues. (Please note that this is a very complex issue, so you are getting the summary version here).

As the HPA Axis is constantly overstimulated from stress, the Adrenal Dysfunction progresses into later stages, and the cortisol levels will eventually fall (or "flatline") because the body can't produce enough cortisol, along with other related issues.

Six Natural Ways to Improve Energy

No matter what the reason for your low energy, these methods can help. (Be sure to talk to a Functional Medicine practitioner to get more specific advice.)

- *Hydration*
- *Movement*
- *Sleep*
- *De-Stress*
- *Green Tea*
- *Eat 6-9 Colors of Vegetables & Fruits a Day*

Hydration: Drink your water! It's essential for blood flow, which transports oxygen around your body for energy. Try coconut water for extra electrolytes. LIMIT or avoid caffeine.

Movement/Physical activity: Move that glorious body of yours! Dance even if you have no rhythm—just move! Get at least ten minutes daily. Find the best time that works for you. Physical activity lowers the stress response and improves mood. It's also been shown to keep you motivated on your health journey.[8]

Rainbow Colored Diet: Shoot for every color of the rainbow each day, nine to thirteen servings. Real food is food that is able to rot. Yes—rot! If it can rot, that means it's loaded with vitamins, minerals, and enzymes. Obviously, you don't want to eat it after it rots, but you do want to eat food that is able to rot. When you're under stress, B vitamins and vitamin C, found in real food, are depleted. You can also increase moisture-rich foods such as kale and spinach for hydration support. Limit or avoid inflammatory-type foods such as gluten and dairy.

Sleep: This is a catch-22 because if you don't get enough sleep, your body will throw off the cortisol rhythm during the day (hello fatigue!)... and irregular cortisol rhythm causes extreme difficulty in falling and staying asleep. You can take some herbs and amino acids to suppress the cortisol at night and possibly raw adrenal to increase it in the mornings, depending on your symptoms or cortisol tests. For raw adrenal, it's always best to test first.

De-stress: Remove things from your life that are not essential and people from your life that are toxic. Let go of what you can't control.

Green Tea: Freshly made green tea (NOT the kind from a can or bottle!) contains epigallocatechin gallate (ECGC), which feeds your cell mitochondria, your energy powerhouse. Drink two cups of freshly brewed green tea a day.

---

8   Den'etsu Sutoo and Kayo Akiyama, "Regulation of Brain Function by Exercise," *Neurobiology of Disease* 13, no. 1 (June 2003): 1–14, https://doi.org/10.1016/S0969-9961(03)00030-5.

Digestive Issues

80 percent of your body's immune system is located in your gut, so if you don't have a healthy gut, it's unlikely you have a healthy immune system.

In our gastrointestinal tract lining, three important organ systems are embedded: our immune system, our nervous system, and our enteric endocrine system.

If You Want to Fix Your Health, Start with Your Gut

Many people don't realize how much the digestive system affects their health—either positively or negatively.

Your gut wall houses 70-80 percent of your immune cells, which makes sense as this is where your body interfaces with potential toxins from the outside world. You might not attribute digestive issues with arthritis, psoriasis, eczema, headaches/migraines, mood disorders, auto-immune disease (acne, irritable bowel syndrome, chronic fatigue, etc.), autism, allergies, dementia, and cancer. However, many diseases seemingly unrelated to digestive processes actually start with an unhealthy gut.

Your gut performs many jobs nonstop: breaking down food, absorbing nutrients, producing nutrients, and keeping toxins out. That's a load!

FACTS

Your gut cells produce 90-95 percent of your serotonin (natural anti-depressant hormone), and every class of neurotransmitter in your brain also resides in your gut. Anti-depressant medications block serotonin from being destroyed. So, they only recycle it, they don't make it. Heal the gut to increase your serotonin production naturally.

To help it do all those jobs, your gut houses over 500 species and 3 pounds of bacteria. This is your microbiome, and it contributes to weight control, disease prevention, and overall health.

Unfortunately, not all gut flora, or microorganisms that live in your gut, are helpful. If you have too many of the bad types (i.e., yeast/candida, parasites) and not enough of the good types (i.e., those fed by probiotics), then don't even think about weight loss or having a healthy immune system. They just won't happen.

Your "Second Brain"

Did you know your gut is the only organ other than your brain with its own nervous system? It's called the enteric nervous system, and it is our body's communication system, producing many of our neurotransmitters (chemicals transmitting messages through our bodies). Your gut's nervous system acts much like a "second brain." In fact, researchers have found that the gut-brain connection plays an extremely important role in gastrointestinal functioning, and it also plays a role in feeling and intuitive decision-making. "Gut instinct" is real!

Our gut health affects what ends up in our blood, how our hormones are produced, how our nervous system (including the brain) functions, and how our immune system responds. Damage to it affects not just the gut but the whole body. In these cases, dysbiosis/imbalance can appear:

- As IBS (irritable bowel syndrome) or, more seriously, IBD (inflammatory bowel disease) such as Crohn's or ulcerative colitis

- As mood swings and fatigue

- As skin conditions such as eczema, psoriasis, rosacea, acne, or histamine-induced hives

- As stiffness and aching joints
- As anxiety and depression

Questionnaire: How's Your Digestive System?

Do you have gut issues? Some people don't realize when they do. Here are some common signs and symptoms:

_____ I feel fatigued after eating.

_____ I get heartburn.

_____ I have constipation (going less than once a day).

_____ I bloat or have a very full feeling and/or belching, flatulence, or burning right after meals.

_____ I have diarrhea.

_____ I have chronic yeast or fungal infections (vaginal yeast infection, jock itch, athlete's foot, toenail fungus).

_____ I have anal itching.

_____ I have chronic abdominal pains.

_____ I regularly use antacids (acid-blocking drugs, Tums, Maalox, Prilosec, etc.).

_____ I feel nauseated after taking supplements.

_____ I have been diagnosed with food allergies, intolerance, or I seem to have reactions to some things I eat.

_____ I have an intolerance to carbohydrates (eating bread or other sugars causes bloating).

_____ I have excessive stress.

_____ I drink more than three alcoholic beverages a week.

_____ I crave carbs like sweets and bread.

_____ I have sores on my tongue.

_____ I have canker sores.

_____ I have a history of NSAID (ibuprofen, naproxen, etc.) or other anti-inflammatory use.

_____ I have bleeding gums or gingivitis.

_____ I have thrush (whitish tongue).

_____ I have geographic tongue (map-like rash on tongue indicating food allergy or yeast overgrowth).

_____ I frequently use or have frequently used antibiotics in the past (more than one to two times in three years).

_____ I find food that is not fully digested in my stool.

_____ I have greasy, large, poorly formed, foul-smelling stools, or mucus in my stools.

_____ I have a family history of any of the following diseases or conditions:

_____ Rosacea	_____ Acne after adolescence
_____ Autism	_____ Celiac disease (gluten allergy)
_____ ADHD	_____ Eczema
_____ Psoriasis	_____ Chronic autoimmune disease
_____ Chronic hives or urticaria	_____ Inflammatory bowel disease
_____ Chronic fatigue syndrome	_____ Irritable bowel syndrome
_____ Fibromyalgia	

Did you know that reflux medications that are proton-pump inhibitors (PPIs) eventually lead to irritable bowel issues and lower vitamin B12 absorption? MOST reflux issues can easily be resolved without medications by:

- Eating slowly (>20 min) and chewing your food well before swallowing

- Eating a lower carbohydrate diet and limiting acidic foods

- Reducing stress

- Walking after meals

- Using supplements to suppress excess acid production: low dosage melatonin 1mg

- Using supplements to repair and protect the throat: aloe vera, slippery elm, DGL, D-limonene, ginger, Iberogast®, zinc L-carnosine

Medications that can exacerbate reflux are sedatives, narcotics, bisphosphonates, and anticholinergics, along with potassium and iron supplements.

Stress on the HPG Axis

Remember my saying your gut and your brain communicate? Well, your Hypothalamus-Pituitary-Gut (HPG) Axis plays a role in your health. The effect of stress in the brain (hypothalamus-pituitary) plays a role in our gut health via our nervous system. And our gut health can create stress on the brain. It's a cycle...a spiral of events linked together. It could become a nasty cycle, bringing about nervous system issues and a decrease in neurotransmitter production. This puts you at high risk for anxiety, panic attacks, depression, poor quality sleep, etc.

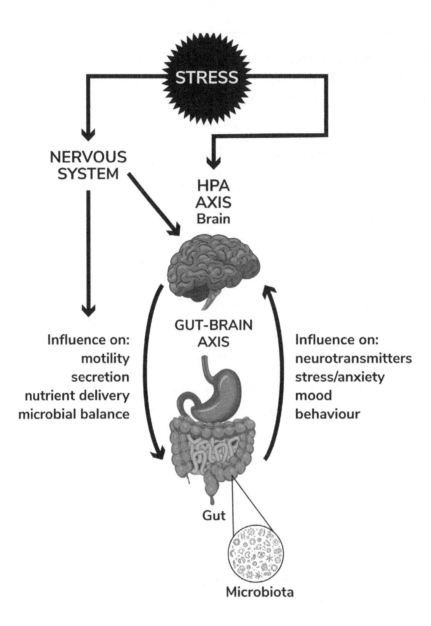

Chronic stress eventually takes a toll on the HPG Axis, including:

- Poor gut motility (constipation, diarrhea)

- Unhealthy gut lining that could lead to food allergy issues, leaky gut syndrome, inadequate neurotransmitter production, low calcium-d-glucarate (needed to decrease estrogen dominance), and decreased short-chain fatty acids in the colon (needed for colon health and cancer prevention), only to name a few

- Killing off the good bacteria lining the gut, leaving more room for bad yeast growth such as candida or SIBO (small intestinal bowel overgrowth)

In summary, the health of your gut plays a critical role in your overall health. Its condition cycles back around to affect your adrenal gland functions and your ability to handle stress, thus affecting your thyroid and sex hormone production.

Tips for Healing Your Gut: A Holistic Functional Medicine Approach

As I've mentioned, instead of managing symptoms with prescription meds, we need to use those symptoms as clues to find and address the root cause that started it all in the first place.

When patients come to me with gut issues, this is the order in which we work together to incorporate the "Four Rs" of healing:

REMOVE processed, sugar-loaded foods; remove "bad bugs" (or bad gut flora), drugs, and allergy-causing foods.

REPLACE unhealthy foods with healthy live food, as well as needed enzymes, fiber, and prebiotics.

REINOCULATE the gut-lining microbiome with good bacteria.

REPAIR the damaged gut lining by supplementing food intake with things such as omega-3s, zinc, glutamine, and/or other necessary healing nutrients.

Case Study #6: "Nathan," Teen with Extreme Bowel Issues

Nathan, a nineteen-year-old, had headaches and extreme bowel issues from constipation to diarrhea. He had mucus in his stool, foul-smelling stool, and some stools that contained undigested foods and were blood tinged. He had been admitted into a children's hospital multiple times over his life and had visited numerous specialists, all of whom said he had irritable bowel and possibly food allergies. He and his dad came to me desperately seeking answers. We did a stool test along with a food allergy and sensitivity test.

Diagnosis:

His food allergy and sensitivity test results came back with a lot of items to avoid.

A stool test showed dysbiosis, metabolic imbalance, and inflammation. All of his good bacteria in his intestinal lining (microbiome) were completely wiped out from the antibiotics over the past several years, plus his typical teenager diet wasn't helping.

He had developed a leaky gut and did not have a healthy gut microbiome to properly break down protein and triglycerides. He didn't have sufficient short-chain fatty acids and butyrate for bowel movements. Thankfully, he had no parasites.

Goals:

- Reduce the bad gut flora

- Reduce his food intolerances/sensitivity

- Repair the gut microbiome

Treatment:

- New diet of non-processed, higher fiber foods, avoiding the allergy/intolerance foods

- Prebiotics and probiotics

- Some plant tannin supplements to kill off the bad bacteria

- Slippery elm supplement for mucosal support

Three Months Later: Nathan was a completely different young man! He was able to hold down a job and go to college without fear of living in the bathroom or fear of food, making him double over in pain.

"I've been in pain since I was pregnant with my last child. My doctor said I have rheumatoid arthritis. How can a thirty-four-year-old have arthritis already? My mom had it, but she didn't get it until she was fifty-four.

Well, I did what you said and cleaned up my diet and took the supplements. I can't believe how much of a difference those simple changes made in only four weeks. And who would have thought foods from the nightshade family would have been a big issue for me? Not only is my arthritis going away, but I'm seeing differences in other areas. I don't ache when I get out of bed each morning nor bloat anymore after meals. There's no more need for laxative at all—I go like clockwork! I do miss drinking all my coffee, but I'm doing ok on one cup a day; it's not killing me to have just one. And I have not had a migraine since I started on this. I've told my mom about you. She wants to come see you too!" —*Shelley, Arkansas*

CHAPTER 8

Inflammation— More Common than You Think

Current health information sources toss buzzwords like "inflammation" around a lot. But what exactly IS inflammation?

I'm sure you've heard of eczema, high blood pressure, hives, rheumatoid arthritis, and swollen ankles...but did you know they are types of inflammation?

Inflammation is the body's healthy response to injury or acute infection. With an infection, your body creates an inflammatory response to accelerate healing. Inflammatory responses are healthy, but they become problematic when they don't go away after a threat subsides or if they show back up when there's no real threat at all. This is called chronic inflammation, which is one of the main underlying causes of many common symptoms and conditions, such as arthritis or autoimmune disorders. It shows up in the form of pain, fatigue, or mood swings as well.

Are you curious whether you have inflammation? See if you have any of these issues:

_____ I have seasonal or environmental allergies.

_____ I have food allergies or sensitivities, or I don't feel well after eating (brain fog, sluggishness, headaches, confusion, etc.)

_____ I have dermatitis (eczema, acne, hives, rashes).

_____ I am overweight and have a hard time losing weight.

_____ I get frequent colds and infections.

_____ I work in an environment with poor lighting, chemicals, and/or poor ventilation.

_____ I am exposed to pesticides, toxic chemicals, loud noise, heavy metals, and /or toxic people in my life (bosses, coworkers, family members).

_____ I have a family history of colitis or inflammatory bowel disease.

_____ I have a family history of diabetes.

_____ I drink more than three glasses of alcohol a week.

_____ I suffer from arthritis.

_____ I have a family history of autoimmune disease (rheumatoid arthritis, lupus, hypothyroidism, etc.)

_____ I have a family history of bronchitis or asthma.

_____ I have a family history of irritable bowel syndrome (spastic colon).

_____ I have a history of chronic infections such as hepatitis, skin infections, canker sores, and/or cold sores.

_____ I have had a heart attack or have a family history of heart disease.

_____ I have sinusitis and allergies.

_____ I have mood and behavior problems.

_____ I have a family history of Parkinson's or Alzheimer's.

_____ I have a stressful life.

_____ I don't exercise for more than thirty minutes, three times a week.

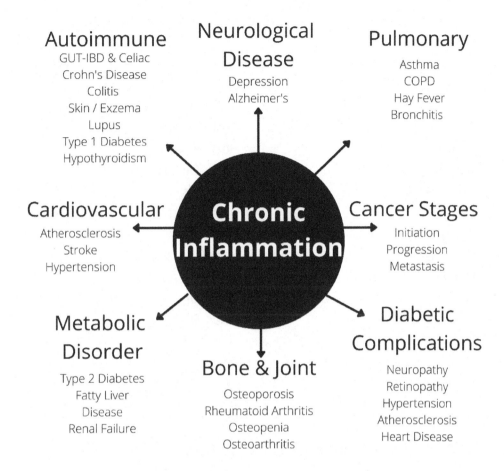

Chronic inflammation can have many causes: Standard American Diet (SAD diet), immune deficiency, long-term physical or emotional stress, poor quality/ insufficient sleep, or even physical injury, just to name a few. The biggest of all the causes is the SAD diet.

As you can see in the diagram above, there's a reason why "inflammation" is one of the buzzwords. It affects multiple body systems. Once you have inflammation, it acts much like a forest wildfire with flames spreading easily.

Some clients initially come to me for weight loss. After looking through their Nutrition Intake Form, which they turn in before our first session, I can assess the healing we have to do to calm those inflammation flames FIRST before any weight loss can occur. For weight loss to occur, we have to get to the root cause. Inflammation stands in the way of weight loss every time.

If you experience any of these symptoms, you are dealing with inflammation:

Acne	Gut Issues (leaky gut, chronic
Alzheimer's	peptic ulcer, ulcerative colitis,
Anxiety	Crohn's disease)
Arthritis	Headaches
Asthma	Heart Disease
Autoimmune Disease	Hepatitis
Brain Fog	Hives/Histamine Intolerances
Cough/Congestion	Irritable Bowel Syndrome
Depression	Joint Pain or Stiffness
Diabetes	Mood Swings
Eczema/Psoriasis	Periodontitis
Environmental Allergies	Sinus Problems
Fatigue	Skin Rash
Fibromyalgia	Weight Gain
Food Allergies	

Food Plays a Major Role in Inflammation

As I mentioned, the SAD diet plays the most significant role in inflammation. Sugar and acidic foods/drinks have the most profound effect. But there's more too, that play a role:

- Artificial colors (found in juice, powdered drink mixes, candy, etc.)

- Artificial preservatives

- Artificial sweeteners (i.e., Splenda®, Sweet'N Low®, Equal®, aspartame)

- Deep-fried foods

- Excess alcohol (beer and wine, but especially hard liquor)

- Excess caffeine (coffee, tea, energy drinks)

- Food allergies:

  ○ The number one food allergy in America is gluten.

  ○ Number two is dairy.

  ○ Other allergy- or sensitivity-producing foods are corn, nuts, eggs, soy, fish/shellfish, or baker's yeast.

  ○ Foods from the nightshade family also seem to be a problem for many people, especially those with rheumatoid arthritis (tomatoes, eggplant, peppers, potatoes).

- Hydrogenated oils such as margarine or any prepackaged baked goods with an extended shelf life

- MSG (monosodium glutamate)

Studies estimate that close to 77 percent of inflammatory reactions are determined by factors we can control, including our diets. The remainder is determined by genetics.

What we choose to eat sends our body signals, influencing how we feel on a daily basis. In the long-term, each bite of food or drink makes the difference between being unhealthy or healthy. So yes, every bite counts.

Pain and fatigue are the number one reasons people seek medical care.

The Center for Disease Control (CDC) stated in 2018 that chronic pain contributes to an estimated $560 billion each year in direct medical costs, lost productivity, and disability programs.

James Dahlhamer, Jacqueline Lucas, Carla Zelaya, and additional contributors, "Prevalence of Chronic Pain and High-Impact Chronic Pain Among Adults," *Morbidity and Mortality Weekly Report* 67, no. 36 (September 2018): 1001–1006.

How to Fight Inflammation

Change your food choices. There is no cookie-cutter "best" specific diet because our biochemistry is so individualized. The foods that work great for a friend might not work well for you. Based on the situation, I like to take combinations of several routes with my clients to eliminate inflammation:

1. **Anti-Inflammatory Program (SHAPE ReClaimed):** This program I offer removes ALL known foods that cause allergy issues. Along with the program, I usually pair inflammation-fighting supplements and other methods to get to the root cause much more quickly. In the last phases of the program, my client starts to add foods back in slowly and can almost immediately experience body issues in the joints or stomach when a new food is reintroduced back into the daily intake. Every one of them loses weight quickly, too, as a byproduct of decreased inflammation.

2. **Elimination Diet:** this is exactly what it sounds like; we use the process of elimination to determine which foods create a reaction in the body. This route can be frustrating for some because it takes weeks to months to figure out if the body is having issues with a food or not.

3. **Food Allergy Test:** I often recommend tests via blood sample to determine food sensitivities, intolerance, and allergies. This gives immediate information on which foods create inflammation.

It's also important to mention to try to eat half of a plate of low carbohydrate/low glycemic foods at each meal with lots of colors, which offers phytonutrients, vitamins, and minerals. Try to eat at least nine different colors of vegetables and fruits a day. If you are not a vegetarian, about one-fourth of your plate should be lean proteins. The last one-fourth should be divided out. Take a small sliver out for plant fats. The last of that one-fourth should be your higher carb "whole" foods such as clean grains (quinoa, oats, brown/wild rice), starchy vegetables (beans, peas, potatoes, corn), fruit, and milk.

Other Ways to Fight Inflammation (Reduce Oxidative Stress):

Meditate, or do yoga and deep diaphragmatic breathing. These calm the nervous system, thus calming the stress reaction, thus calming the oxidative inflammatory response. Research even shows it makes the body more stress resilient.

All it takes is five minutes a day to make a difference. Research studies have shown that meditation can help decrease inflammation.

Yoga releases stored tension and heavy energy created from inflammatory oxidative stress.

> Stress Resiliency is the acquired ability to meet life's challenges (stressors), bounce back from challenging experiences, and become more capable and confident as a result.

Stimulate the vagus nerve.[9] This nerve, which is the "communication highway from the brain to the gut," also branches off to the liver, heart, and lungs. Stimulating it—which you can do by slow deep belly breathing, singing, or deep belly humming—has been shown to lower inflammation in clients with rheumatoid arthritis, as well as alleviate inflammation-related health issues such as depression and inflammatory bowel disease.

Get seven to nine hours of quality sleep. I'll go into a lot of detail on sleep in the next chapter. For the time being, just know that sleep not only helps us feel optimal, but it also combats unhealthy levels of inflammation.[10] In fact, just a two-hour nap has been shown to significantly lower inflammation levels that were elevated from lack of sleep the night before.

Try intermittent fasting (IF). Intermittent fasting is an eating pattern in which a person fasts during some periods and eats during others, with the fasting period usually longer than the "eating window." This allows the body to rest, without having to digest foods, for longer periods of time. It has been linked to a decrease in inflammation-related health conditions like asthma, lupus, dementia, and IBS. Please talk to your doctor before doing this! Some people will NOT benefit from it due to other health issues involved.

---

9   Frieda A. Koopman, Sangeeta S. Chavan, Sanda Miljko, Simeon Grazio, Sekib Sokolovic, P. Richard Schuurman, Ashesh D. Mehta, Yaakov A. Levine, Michael Faltys, Ralph Zitnik, Kevin J. Tracey, and Paul P. Tak, "Vagus Nerve Inhibits Cytokine Production and Attenuates Disease Severity in Rheumatoid Arthritis," *PNAS* 13, no. 29 (July 2016): 8284 –8289. https://doi.org/10.1073/pnas.1605635113.

10 Elsevier, "Loss of Sleep, Even for a Single Night, Increases Inflammation in the Body," ScienceDaily, September 4, 2008, Accessed June 30, 2020 from www.sciencedaily.com/ releases/2008/09/080902075211.htm.

Increase a protein called Nrf-2. This protein lowers inflammation. You can increase it by consuming the following through antioxidant-rich foods:

- EGCG (epigallocatechin gallate) found in freshly brewed green tea (not a bottled tea)

- Quercetin, found in apples or in a supplement

- Curcumin, from turmeric

- Resveratrol, from grapes or red wine

- Rosmarinic, acid from rosemary

- L-sulforaphane, from broccoli or even better, broccoli sprouts

- Thiosulfonateallicin, from garlic

- Omega-3s, from wild-caught fish or taking omega-3 supplements (fish oils)[11] or plant-based omegas such as flax seeds, chia seeds, or walnuts.

- Vitamin C, as found in citrus[12],[13]

Once your "firefighting" approach helps cool down the inflammation "flames," your body can start healing—and of course, the byproduct is losing the unwanted weight. Until then, inflammation will block the body's natural ability to heal and balance.

---

11 Han Li, Xiong Z. Ruan, Stephen H. Powis, David C. Wheeler, John F. Moorhead, and Zac Varghese, "EPA and DHA Reduce LPS-Induced Inflammation Responses in HK-2 Cells: Evidence for a PPAR-Gamma-Dependent Mechanism." Kidney International 67, no. 3 (March 2005):867-874. https://doi.org/10.1111/j.1523-1755.2005.00151.x.

12 Michel Langlois, Daniel Duprez, Joris Delanghe, Marc De Buyzere, and Denis L. Clement, "Serum Vitamin C Concentration Is Low in Peripheral Arterial Disease and Is Associated with Inflammation and Severity of Atherosclerosis," Circulation 103 (April 2001):1863–1868. https://doi.org/10.1161/01.CIR.103.14.1863.

13 S. Goya Wannamethee, Gordon DO Lowe, Ann Rumley, K. Richard Bruckdorfer, and Peter H. Whincup, "Associations of Vitamin C Status, Fruit and Vegetable Intakes, and Markers of Inflammation and Hemostasis," *The American Journal of Clinical Nutrition* 83, no. 3 (March 2006):567–727. http://doi.org/10.1093/ajcn.83.3.567.

More Food Tips

By now, you probably realize that nutrition is a foundation for good health. Making good food choices can make a big difference, not only in fighting inflammation, but in helping your body heal and prevent multiple issues naturally. Since choosing the right food is so important, I want to give you some tips.

Make Good Nutritional Choices

The "Bad, Good, Better, Best" chart can help you look at your food choices wisely and make changes where needed.

Also, keep in mind how processed your food is. If it's grown from the ground or picked from a tree, consider it good. If it's from a box, can, package, or factory, has artificial ingredients, or has an extended shelf life, then it is man-made or man-manipulated and lacks quality. In other words, it's not a healthy choice.

Many have found a plant-based diet helps fight inflammation, but it's imperative to still avoid processed plant-based "food products."

You don't have to shop at high-end health food stores to get your necessities either. You can go to any local grocery store to get your basics. Eating healthy, real food needs to be kept simple, or you're less likely to do it.

BAD ▶ GOOD ▶ BETTER ▶ BEST

PRINCIPLE

"Doing the best you can with what you have"

*GMO = Genetically modified organisms. Genetic material has been altered using genetic engineering which will destroy all or decrease nutritious value (e.g. corn and soy).

	BAD	GOOD	BETTER	BEST
VEGETABLES & FRUITS	Not eating ANY fresh fruits or vegetables	Buying only conventional fruits & vegetables	Using the Dirty Dozen or Clean Fifteen Rule & buying organic	All organic, local and seasonal, &/or growing your own
GRAINS & FLOURS	Quick fix packaged cereals, chips, crackers, granola bars, poptart & snack foods	Homemade cooking with some refined flours or GMO loaded flours	Homemade cooking with 100% "whole" grains & flours	Homemade cooking with 100% "whole" grains. Preparing properly by soaking, sprouting, or sour leavening
EGGS	Eating egg whites only, powdered eggs, or egg-like products	Buying conventional store-bought cheaper eggs	Buying store-bought organic, free-range eggs	Buying organic & local pasture-raised eggs
DAIRY (milk, cheese)	Low-fat dairy products, high-temperature pasteurized, from cows given hormones/steroids	Whole or 2% dairy, primarily grass-fed & low-temperature pasteurized	Whole or 2% dairy, primarily grass-fed &/or raw	Whole or 2% primarily pasture-raised, organic & raw, from cows never given hormones/steroids
MEAT (turkey, chicken, beef, pork)	Boneless, from animals given antibiotics &/or hormones/ steroids, processed	Non-processed, antibiotic & hormone free	Non-processed, grass-fed, &/or organic	Non-processed, primarily grass-fed &/ or organic, pasture-raised (not corn or other GMO-loaded-grain fed)
SEAFOOD	GMO or seafood-like processed products	Farm-raised seafood, BPA-lined canned	BPA-free canned or frozen wild caught seafood	Fresh & local wild caught seafood
FATS	Margarine, shortening, soybean oil, corn oil, canola oil, vegetable oil & hydrogenated oils	Pasteurized store-bought grain-fed butter	Pasteurized organic grass-fed butter OR regular coconut/olive/ avocado oil	Grass-fed lard & tallow OR organic, extra-virgin coconut or olive oil, avocado oil, ghee, or raw butter
SWEETENERS	High Fructose Corn Syrup, GMO white sugar, sugar substitutes (e.g. Splenda®, Sweet 'n Low®, Equal ®, etc)	100% pure unrefined cane sugar	Store bought, honey, real maple syrup, monk fruit	Local honey, organic unrefined cane sugar, organic real maple syrup, pure stevia, or coconut sugar
PANTRY ITEMS	GMO laden cereals, crackers, chips, snack foods	Organic, non-GMO cereals, crackers, chips, snack foods	Homemade whole grain cereals, crackers, chips, snack foods	Homemade whole grain prepared OR even better, stop recreating them & just go simple and real

CHAPTER 9

Sleep—A Foundational Solution

My husband and I started remodeling our house just three weeks before COVID-19 shut the country down. We built our house when we were young pups twenty years before, choosing whatever was on sale because we were broke but needed a bigger house since baby number two was on the way. When I say, "on sale," I mean bronze light fixtures with chrome faucets because it was in the bargain bin. It was an interior designer's nightmare, trust me. But we were proud owners, and it was ours.

The main reason for the remodeling was our kitchen (and to finally get the fixtures to all match), which was too small. It had served its purpose over the years of providing dinner for the family, and the kids with their oh-so-cute aprons on, cranking out Christmas cookies. It held many memories of sleepovers and the kids laughing as they created some midnight snack or my son coming up with his next science experiment concoction. It was the gathering place for family and friends, but its size always created a traffic jam. It needed work, and the rest of the house needed a facelift as well.

To open up the room and make it more user-friendly, we wanted the wall separating our kitchen and living room to be removed. This would require an orderly, step-by-step process because that was a supporting wall structure for the floor upstairs. If it was done out of order, the floor upstairs would come crashing down.

To accomplish this huge task, the contractor had to have everything lined up. This wall had to be worked on first before they could proceed to the rest of the house. And they had to make sure the foundation was firm enough to make those major changes.

Isn't that similar to our health? Putting on a fresh coat of paint doesn't fix structural things that are messed up. And we can't start making huge changes when the structure might not be secure. To have a strong structure, you have to have a firm foundation. Your health is no different. Its foundation is the proper nourishment of your Mind-Body-Spirit.

We can't make huge changes in your health without a step-by-step plan to help us arrive safely at the final product we desire; otherwise, our efforts will create other problems, and the entire structure will quickly crumble. This is where I act as your "health contractor" by laying out that step-by-step plan to help you to obtain your goals.

Along with nutrition, one major part of your health foundation is sleep. You may have noticed that sleep has been a part of almost every list of my "health tips." The reason is that your body systems reboot and repair the best during sleep, and sleep also gives you the stamina to deal with stress.

What Sleep Does for Your Health

- Controls weight

- Improves control of blood sugars

- Builds the immune system

- Reboots energy and mood

- Repairs muscle

- Decreases blood pressure (which decreases stroke risk in those with hypertension)

- Sharpens thinking, attention to detail, and emotional awareness

- Decreases inflammation

- Boosts creativity

- Decreases stress

Sleep Reboots Hormones, Metabolism, Nervous System

If you have ever felt drained or foggy after a poor night's sleep, it shouldn't surprise you that sleep significantly impacts your brain function, energy, metabolism, and resetting the nervous system. You need sleep to handle stress better!

"Brain plasticity," or the ability to adapt to input (learning), is compromised with poor sleep. Why didn't someone bring this to my attention back in college?

Sleep is vital to the whole body. Lack of sleep increases health risks. Those horrible symptoms of anxiety, depression, high blood pressure, seizures, and migraines/headaches worsen. Sleep also helps with brain "cleanup," or getting rid of toxins.[14] Have you ever noticed that your immune system goes south when you don't get enough sleep?

You want to lose weight? Get sleep!

Sleep plays a role in metabolism: Even one night of missed sleep can increase HPA-Axis Dysfunction, decrease motivation, and increase the risk of a pre-diabetic state in an otherwise healthy person.

Processes of Sleep: Circadian Rhythms

Circadian rhythms are controlled by the brain's biological clock. One of its key functions is to respond to light cues, increasing production of the hormone melatonin at night, then switching it off when it senses light. This is why you should try to sleep in a dark room and turn off all screens (TV, phone, iPad, Kindle, computer, etc.) an hour before bed to prime the body to make melatonin.

---

14 Björn Rasch and Jan Born, ⬚About Sleep⬚s Role in Memory,⬚ *Physiological Reviews* 93, no. 2 (April 2013):681–766. https://doi.org/10.1152/physrev.00032.2012.

I often have to run tests on clients to assess the patterns in their melatonin and cortisol production. Balancing the circadian rhythm is crucial; otherwise, the chances of anxiety and panic attacks greatly increase.

How Much Sleep Do We Need?

Research shows we need seven to nine hours of uninterrupted sleep to reap all the health benefits. Ayurveda Medicine[15] research says that the hours of 10 p.m. to 2 a.m. are the best hours of sleep for rebooting. (Ayurvedic medicine is a natural system of medicine that originated in India more than three thousand years ago.)

Tips for Better-Quality Sleep

Minimize or Avoid Stimulants

- Avoid alcohol within three hours of bedtime.

- Avoid caffeine-containing beverages or foods after 2 p.m.

- Avoid cold medicines containing pseudoephedrine or other similar decongestants (which act as stimulants) at night.

- Avoid aerobic-type exercise at least four hours before bed.

Nighttime, Right Before Bedtime

- Avoid anxiety-provoking activities (watching news or catching up on social media).

- Avoid paying bills or checking financial reports or the stock market before bed because it gets the brain thinking!

- Plan your schedule for eight-and-a-half to nine hours of sleep, even if you wake up after seven hours.

---

15 Suhas Kshirsagar and Michelle D. Seaton, *Change Your Schedule, Change Your Life* (New York: Harper Wave, 2018).

- Begin getting ready for bed at least thirty minutes before bedtime (washing your face, brushing your teeth, taking a bath, etc.).

- Avoid large meals before bed and try to finish eating at least three hours or longer before bedtime.

- Avoid drinking more than six ounces of fluid right before bed. Who likes getting up to pee in the middle of the night?

- Take a hot Epsom salts bath (one to two cups salt) with aroma-therapy, such as lavender essential oil, before bed. This can raise your body temperature, helping to induce sleep while dropping your cortisol levels. The heat and the magnesium from the Epsom salt absorbing into your skin also relax the muscles and reduce tension. Another alternative is adding a half to a full cup of baking soda in the bath to alkalize a stressed-out, acidic body.

- Drink a calming (herbal) tea such as chamomile or one formulated to help with sleep.

- Keep your mobile devices, computers, and other distractions either out of the room or away from the bed.

Strategies to Use with Trouble Falling Asleep

- Try red light therapy. There've been lots of recent studies on this showing how it improves production of melatonin.

- Don't stay in bed for more than thirty minutes trying to fall asleep. Leave your bedroom and relax in another room using a relaxation technique (meditate, listen to brainwave music, read from a real [not electronic!] book, etc.).

- If you must use a tablet or phone for reading, make sure it is in the nighttime setting, with the brightness as low as possible.

- Put dark coverings over the windows to cut out all light.

- Keep your bedroom colder, even if you have to sleep naked under heavy covers. A colder room helps most people to fall asleep more easily.

- Use a weighted blanket.

- Decrease irritating noises in your bedroom, even if you need a white noise generator.

Supplements that Could Help with Sleep

Remember—each person has a unique biochemistry, so not all of these will work the same way for everyone. This is not meant to be medical advice for you, but just an idea of what things I might prescribe. Get advice from your medical practitioner before you start taking supplements.

- Melatonin: 1–5 mg to fall asleep and/or 5–20 mg time-release melatonin to stay asleep. This should not be used nightly—only as needed.

- 5-HTP: 100–200 mg one hour before bed (you should NOT take this if on a prescription antidepressant). Works best if you take B-complex and vitamin C.

- L-Theanine: Boosts GABA and other calming brain chemicals. It elevates serotonin and dopamine and helps lower anxiety and stress.

- Taurine: 500–2000 mg one hour before bed.

- Magnesium: 200–600 mg in split doses (e.g., 200 mg morning, 400 mg evening).

- GABA: 100–200 mg one hour before bed. Helps parasympathetic activity go up.

- Vitamin B6: 100-300 mg/day with food.

- To decrease nighttime cortisol or stress, consider adaptogens (ashwagandha, valerian root, holy basil, passionflower, rhodiola) with calming amino acids (phosphatidylserine, L-theanine).

- Establish an evening herbal tea habit (hot or cold), such as lemon balm, passionflower, or chamomile.

- Consider getting a half hour of exposure to a blue or 10,000 lux bright light (first thing in the morning) if you are going to bed too late and want to shift to an earlier bedtime.

Other Calming Strategies for the Body

- Brainwave or bilateral music: Listen to this type of music throughout the day or just in the evening. My favorites are from Dr. Jeffrey Thompson, a neuroacoustic scientist for NASA. He offers brainwave music for de-stressing, self-regulation, and rejuvenating sleep on YouTube.

- Meditation: Research studies have shown that meditation decreases blood pressure, reduces stress, and brings about self-awareness so less emotional eating occurs. I suggest guided meditation apps. My favorite app is called "Insight Timer."

CHAPTER 10

Overcoming Obstacles

What Matters Most?

Have you heard the Bible story about this guy named Peter who stepped off a boat and walked out onto the water? There were storms all around him, waves tossing...but he saw this amazing guy, Jesus, walking on water, and so Peter stepped out towards him. But then, Peter took his eyes off his focus, allowed the storms and waves (and his fear and disbelief in what he was doing) to distract him, and he immediately started sinking.

Aren't we like that in so many ways? We have a goal in mind, but then we get distracted by the storms of life around us: kids demanding attention with homework, work deadlines, a spouse who gives us a weird, disapproving look when we fix a somewhat healthy meal, laundry that has been backed up for days, a sudden pandemic rocking our world...you get my drift? We lose sight of our focus, our goal, within the chaos life throws at us.

I may not be able to walk on water, but my passion is to walk alongside you, to be a guide in helping you reach your goal. And when you lose focus or motivation or belief in yourself, I can help. I'm a firm believer that we have to take small steps, only looking at the one step in front of us and not looking at the whole long set of stairs we have to climb. We will get there, one step at a time.

Sometimes, the obstacles seem external, but they also have an internal aspect. To be in charge of your health, you have to make different choices, and that means sometimes you might also have to think differently. That includes thinking your way around the blocks that are in your way or the ideas that are letting you drift away from your goals. If any of the following reasons are getting in your way, you're not alone. I've heard a lot of these from my patients. Together, we've worked to get through or around them.

Old Childhood Habits: "I Was Made to Clean My Plate"

One client, who battled with a poor food relationship, told me that it was ingrained in him to "clean his plate," or eat everything on it, since childhood. He knew it was an unhealthy act and did not want his kids battling the same issue, so he didn't make his kids clean their plates. Instead, he did it for them.

As a kid, I was made to clean my plate before I got up from the table a well. At one point, I sat at the table for two hours because I did not want to put liver in my mouth. As an adult, breaking this pattern of "cleaning my plate" had to be intentional. Our upbringing becomes so ingrained in us that we don't realize the habits we learned could sometimes be destructive. Overconsuming or ignoring fullness cues only destroys the efforts of improving health.

We are not a human trash can.

I totally understand the reasoning behind the "clean your plate" philosophy...it all stems from the Great Depression. But we are no longer in the Great Depression. We can cover up food left on our plate and come back to it later when we are hungry again—developing a better relationship with food by noticing our patterns and questioning if they are truly healthy.

"I Can't Afford the Money/Time"

I hear people voice this concern often. Some of the things that trigger this response are:

- **Insurance.** If their insurance doesn't cover alternative treatment or doesn't cover everything needed, they can be concerned about paying the costs out of pocket.

- **Additional testing.** Even if insurance does cover all the testing needed, doing more lab tests than conventional medicine creates a higher upfront cost. (Possibly, but not everyone needs extra testing. And if testing is necessary, it will provide valuable information that can assist in a regimen to speed up healing.)

- **The idea that healthy choices = additional cost.** Many people feel organic food is too expensive, or that buying produce, etc., is more expensive than their favorite easy processed meals. (I can easily show you this is not true. And it is not necessary to purchase all organic. Just take a peek at the end of this chapter and the "Bad-Good-Better-Best" chart in chapter 8).

- **Gyms are too expensive.** Many feel they have to be a member of a gym in order to exercise. This is far from true. A good pair of walking shoes is a great start for non-gym workouts. Swimming, hiking, biking, or doing body-weight training, such as air squats or wall pushups, are great sources of movement at home!

- **Hectic lifestyle.** Often, people don't feel they have time to think about cooking or focus on nutritional planning. While not a monetary cost, time is precious to most of us—and we never seem to have enough of it. I get it. But small tweaks in lifestyle will start you towards better health. And remember what the Dalai Lama said about spending our lives trying to increase wealth, only to have to spend our wealth all on our poor health. Let's change this perspective!

I'm willing to pay cash if my insurance won't cover the consultation. I don't want a bandage. I want an answer and cure. —*Marsha, Searcy, Arkansas*

Being Unhealthy Costs More Money than You Realize

If any of the above costs are something you're worried about, I understand. However, I'd like to challenge you for a minute to think differently.

Remember when you added all the financial costs of your poor health? How much are you already paying to be unhealthy? And have you thought about the hidden costs you maybe aren't even adding up, or what you would save if you weren't paying ANY of those costs?

Hmmm. That changes the perspective, doesn't it?

Here's an example of the hidden costs of poor health. A few years back, my family and I flew to Colorado for some time on the slopes during my kids' Christmas break. We booked it last minute, so our seats were scattered on the plane. I was hoping to possibly trade seats with someone to be close to my youngest one before takeoff. I noticed there was an empty seat across the aisle from where my youngest sat. From behind, where I was, the seat next to the empty seat looked to be taken by a man. The backside of his head had greyish-white hair that was receding. I walked toward the front of the plane, approaching the balding man sitting next to the window. As I began to ask, "Do you mind if I sit here?" my heart quickly moved up to my throat as if to cut off my words in mid-sentence. He was a man whose obesity required him to raise the middle armrest so that he could occupy one-and-a-half seats. I assume he had paid for both to accommodate his larger size. I will never forget his worn-out, glassy blue eyes looking up at me. What I saw in them was so much heartache, brokenness, and loss of hope. I could see that he had a sense of what I had meant to ask him and that the wheels in his mind were turning and thinking, "How do I explain why I have to decline your request...is it not that obvious that you can't sit down beside me?" Being an empath, I immediately felt the heaviness he carried within from his life experiences that had brought him to this point of hopelessness. It absolutely broke my heart. I will never forget that plane trip, nor that man.

From a financial perspective, poor health will cost you more than prevention. In the case of the older gentleman, it was the cost of paying for two seats, and it could have cost him the embarrassment of explaining why I couldn't sit down.

It's a tough thing to think about. But you need to care about yourself enough to ask yourself, in the greater picture of life, what is truly worth it? You can pay a little now or pay for it—maybe a lot more—later.

Here are just some of the potential ways you might already be "paying later":

- Buying two plane seats instead of one on every flight

- Paying more for, and spending more time hunting for, plus-sized clothing

- Paying for all your prescription medications each month (remember to multiply that cost over the rest of your entire life)

- Paying for hospital stays or specialized medical treatments and equipment you may not have needed if you were in better health preventatively

- Lost work due to chronic or serious illness

- Lost family time due to just not feeling well enough to participate in events or be fully engaged in relationships

Here's another example.

You can take a couple of hours out of your week to cook several meals ahead or to prep food to make cooking easier throughout the week

OR

you can go the easiest route by just going through a fast-food drive-through.

The first one:
1. saves you money long-term because it's always cheaper to cook at home and

2. feeds your health preventatively now, saving money on health expenses in the future.

Meanwhile, the other one:
- saves you time at that very moment, but ends up being very costly over the long term by doing it at every meal and

- feeds your body the SAD diet, which, as we've seen, causes inflammation, leading eventually to chronic health issues that will set your health and your bank account back in the long run.

> "I've always said I'd never eat a diabetic diet if I got diabetes. Well, here I am with diabetes and heart disease. You made it so easy to understand, which made it easier for me to follow. My HgbA1c is down from 12 to 5.3 now! And my cholesterol has dropped from 236 down to 183. My coworkers are asking me what diet I'm on and I've learned to reply, 'I'm not on a diet, only a lifestyle change.' You've made my wife happy because of how much this has changed me for the better. We have started walking in the evenings together too, and even got our kids to ride the bikes alongside us, so it's actually been a good change for our family." —*Robert, Texas*

"I Want Quicker Results."

Years ago, before my last child was born, I worked in a hospital. One of the new patients on my floor was a gastric bypass patient that was sent over from the nursing home because she was having some difficulties from the gastric bypass surgery. As always, I looked through the chart to gather pertinent information about the patient's needs before I went into the room. I noticed that this patient was twenty-nine years old. This has to be a typo, I thought. I read further, and it repeated the age of twenty-nine again. So, I asked one of the nurses if there was a mix-up. Come to find out, she WAS twenty-nine years old! She had had a gastric bypass that went bad, and neither she nor her family could take care of her needs, so she lived in a nursing home to get the right medical care.

I went in to talk to her about some lifestyle changes in small steps that could help her out. We briefly went over better food choices—modified in form to meet the demands of the gastric bypass issues—along with recommendations for some liquid multivitamins and minerals that could benefit her nourishment. I didn't go over too much because from her chart, she would most likely be in the hospital for a while, and I didn't want to overwhelm her too much on the first visit. She welcomed the information but also seemed like a nervous wreck about her decision, admitting the gastric bypass choice was a bad mistake. She just thought that the easy drive-through fast-food habits would be too hard to break, so the gastric bypass was the easiest option to reach her goals. But as she teared up, she said if she had the chance to do it all over again, she would not have chosen the "easy way out" because it wasn't worth it.

The next Monday, when I got back to work, I found out that the twenty-nine-year-old, who had had a full life ahead of her, had passed away the night before.

All I could hear was her voice telling me that previous Friday that she wished she had never taken the easy route—which ended up not being easy at all.

We need to stop thinking "instant pot" and start thinking "slow cooker"—progress that will last long after the last page is turned. We walk through the progress together.

With each step on your healing journey, you are putting healthy "tools" in your tool belt and learning new ways of doing things to equip you for life's challenges that will inevitably pop up.

The goal isn't just to gain back your health...**it's to gain mental stamina and endurance along with knowledge and foresight.**

There are no shortcuts to any place worth going to.

And you should know by now that if the quick fixes sound too good to be true, that's because yes, they are!

If you asked my clients how long it took them to start feeling some changes or start feeling better, each one of them would tell you that within a few days they could feel a difference. And as each week progressed, they kept improving. How could they NOT improve if they were fueling and nourishing the body the right way? Of course, if you address the root cause (the upstream issue), a multitude of symptoms will start to dissipate (all the downstream ripple effects).

Good health is a long-term investment.
Thinking about health should be as investment, not "cost." You aren't just throwing your money away; you are investing in yourself.

"My Family Will Never Do Things This New Way"

I get it—your partner will only eat mac and cheese, bread, and meat. You like the active lifestyle, and your spouse prefers to sit and watch TV. But that doesn't mean you have to give up meeting your health goals!

1. **YOU DO YOU.** Plain and simple. So far, you've let marketing ads and commercials control you, insurance dictate to you, your busy lifestyle sidetrack you, work stress overwhelm you...isn't it time YOU DO YOU? I'm not by any means suggesting you turn your back on your partner. What I'm saying is, it's time you start doing some self-care for YOU in regard to Mind-Body-Spirit healing, and that means prioritizing yourself as important.

2. **Let others do themselves.** Invite your partner to join you in making some changes for the better but avoid having unreasonable expectations. Have an honest talk with them and ask about their health goals and motivations. If they don't feel ready to make changes, discover why.

    Though you might think your partner needs a diet overhaul, if they aren't ready, they aren't ready. Pushing them only leads to friction. Plus, you never know—your new habits might eventually start to rub off on your reluctant partner.

3. **Establish healthy boundaries.** This will come in handy whether going solo or not. Keep certain areas of the house (like a drawer or refrigerator in the garage) where your partner can stash their junk food where it will be out of your sight. Discuss grocery shopping expectations and be open with your partner about what you are going to cut and add. Ask your partner to try a new food or recipe you make.

> *"If we don't take control of our environment, it takes control of us."*
>
> *"Whether you realize it or not, what goes on around you has a massive influence on the way you feel and the way you act.*
>
> *By taking leadership of your own life, you can defy outside influences and set your own tone for the day ahead, regardless of whatever or whoever is exerting pressure from the outside."*
> —Tony Robbins

4. **Ask for support if they don't want to participate.** This could be something simple such as not eating cookies around you. Speak up if they are doing things or saying things that they don't realize are affecting you negatively in your progress, such as "I love you just as you are." While they might love you as you are, they don't realize that statement's negative effects on your motivation.

5. **Own your behavior.** You might not always be able to control your surroundings, but you are ultimately in control of what's on the fork that's moving up to your lips, or whether or not you put on those jogging shoes and go out for a quick run.

6. **Change up the ways you enjoy your time together.** If your partner is literally your "partner in crime" in unhealthy habits, find something else to do together. For instance, if you both enjoy munching unhealthy snacks in front of the television, find a new activity you can both enjoy together, such as biking or walking. Or cook healthy meals together and try new recipes you both get to pick.

7. **Lead by example.** Just as you can be affected by your loved one's unhealthy habits, it can also go the other way. They can be positively affected by you.

"I Can Never Be/Do [Insert Comparison Here]."

Comparison kills.

Let that sink in...comparison kills.

Comparison allows lies to come into your thoughts, and if you start to believe them, you will set yourself up for failure.

Comparison is based on ideals instead of reality. Because of that, it can lead to condemnation. Condemnation defeats us.

We don't need condemnation; we need conviction. Conviction can unlock your greatest potential for true, everlasting lifestyle change.

So, if so-and-so, who is always posting on social media, brags about how much weight she has lost, and you notice how much more quickly she's lost it than you have, your self-condemnation will mentally trip you up. We are all biochemically different, which means some lose it faster and some lose it slower.

And all those pyramid companies promising weight loss have abandoned the fact that lifestyle change HAS to be a part of their expensive, non-sustainable products that they promote. So, if so-and-so chick is not making true lifestyle changes along the way, that weight will ALL COME BACK ON fast and then some!

You also have to keep in mind what you're measuring as your "comparison." Is it even a valid measurement?

For instance, suppose you're spending all your time trying to reach a certain weight, which is really just a number. But comparing your own current body weight number to some ideal body weight number doesn't give you a real picture of your progress.

You were not created for Comparison! You. BE. You.

Pound for pound, muscle and fat weigh the same. But if you compared the amount of space each one takes up, you would understand why I do NOT like my clients to ONLY go by scale weight. One pound of fat takes up far more space (such as inches on your waist) than muscle.

When I was seven months pregnant with my second child, my brother-in-law died in an accident. Even though I was a registered dietitian and knew how I should eat, his death affected me hard and tripped me up mentally and emotionally. I turned to food as my "drug of choice" in dealing with my depression. I gained an extra thirty pounds in those last two months of pregnancy. I'm sure I was pushing the envelope of developing gestational diabetes with that much weight.

One year later, after not exercising and continuing to stuff my face in grief, I found myself at the same weight, yet was four sizes bigger than I was before my brother-in-law died. It finally clicked, and I knew I had to get out of that depressive funk. So, I started eating clean again and working out. After six months, my weight had stayed the same, but my size had dropped back down to where I was before my pregnancy. Why? Because I increased muscle and lost body fat. Pound for pound, it was the same weight, but I switched the ratios up!

"But My Willpower Failed Me in the Past!"

It's crucial to set yourself up for success. Willpower alone will never work.

There are lots of ways to think creatively to support your goals—and if you create solutions based on your own unique personality and what motivates you, they will be more likely to work. Set your environment up for success. Do what it takes.

That might mean informing your household that you are making healthier changes and you need their support instead of their nose turned up at healthier food being prepared...or it could require joining in with a walking partner to hold each other accountable...or teaming up with a friend who wants to make changes too, and doing a recipe swap, or even doubling up on your meals and swapping your extras for your friend's (not only giving you more food variety, but saving the time of cooking another meal!).

I have clients come in on a WEEKLY basis to see me just because it keeps them accountable. If that is what it takes, then by all means, let's do it!

> "Being a successful person is not necessarily defined by what you have achieved, but by what you have overcome." —*Fannie Flagg, American actress and author*

Budget Shopping

By now, you know you can't get by me with the excuse, "I can't eat healthy because I can't afford it."

And, you already know that healthy does NOT mean you have to always go to a health-food store. In addition, you can do a lot of smart shopping to give you more bang for your nutrition buck. Think SIMPLE.

Here's a sample of budget shopping in the south central region of the USA. (Prices could vary based on where you might live, so use it as a guide.) It's time we break the stigma of healthy food costing too much.

FOOD	COST PER SERVING	HOW TO PURCHASE IN 2021
Potatoes: Baked potatoes, breakfast potatoes, salads, soups/stews	$0.24-$0.33 per medium potato (3/4 cup) or about $0.49 per pound	A 5-pound bag of Russet potatoes costs about $2.50-$2.75, and a bag **contains 11-13 potatoes.** A 10-pound bag averages $5.
Brown Rice: Side dishes, rice salads, soups/stews	$0.18 per 1/4 cup dry rice	A 5-pound bag costs about $3.32 and **contains 50 servings** (1/4 cup dry is a serving).
Old Fashioned Oats: Hot or cold cereal, granola, crumb toppings for yogurts	$0.13 per 1/2 cup cooked or $0.09 per ounce	A 42-ounce container **(30 servings)** is about $3.33.
Lentils: Salads, soups/stews, and more. Lentils cook quickly without pre-soaking.	$0.10 per ¼ cup dried uncooked (will almost double in size after cooking) or $0.06 per ounce	Buy a 16-ounce bag **(12 servings)** for $0.99-$1.29. Buy a 4-pound bag **(52 servings)** for $4.88.
Frozen Vegetables: Side dishes, soups/ stews	$0.21-$0.25 per 1-cup cooked serving	Buy 12-ounce bags and spend about $0.84-$1.00 per bag **(4 servings per bag).**
Bag of Spinach: Quick salads, egg dishes, soups/stews	$0.77 for a 2-cup serving	A bag **(6 ounces/ 3.5 servings)** of washed spinach leaves is about $2.68.
Tuna: Tuna salads and to serve with gluten-free crackers.	$0.85 for chunk light albacore in water; 6 ounces	A 6-ounce can of solid white albacore in water costs about $1.99; a 6-ounce can of chunk white albacore in water is about $1.39.
Chicken (antibiotic-free)	$1.49 per 3 ounce serving	$5.94 per pound, so about $1.48 per 3 ounce serving **(4 servings after cooked).**

My Favorite Insider Shopping Hacks

When you're buying your groceries, you can make some smart decisions that will stretch your money further than you might expect. Here are some ways to save money and your health at the same time:

- **Buy in bulk.** A bag of apples is much cheaper than individual apples, plus bagged apples are closer to accurate serving sizes. And big bags of dry beans can last a while in the pantry!

- **Have a shopping list** and STICK TO IT. Avoid impulsive buying.

- **Buy it if it's in season** or buy it frozen if not. Fruits and veggies out of season can cost double what they do when they're in season.

- **Use coupons** for healthy foods (though they're hard to find!)!

- **Stop eating out!** Not only is restaurant food expensive, but it's also most likely not as healthy. You don't really know what is going into food that you haven't prepared yourself. And you probably know that if the restaurant is using all-natural or organic ingredients, it's going to be more expensive than the others.

- **Buy meat on the bone** for a cheaper deal; plus, the bone offers more calcium and iron in your meat.

- **Cook double what you need** and freeze the extra for another day.

CHAPTER 11

The Power of Holistic Focus

Spirit and Mind: When the "Ah-Ha" Moment Strikes

Spirituality is about our connection to ourselves, our connection to the world around us, having a sense of a higher power, and a sense of belonging and community. To me personally, it's also about the relationship between me and God, who I call "Big Pappa"...and the love and self-love that springs out of that.

The word "spiritual" originates from the Latin word *spiritus*, meaning "breath of life."[16] The spiritual aspect of Mind-Body-Spirit refers to unseen and often mysterious energy working at a deep level on our spiritual being.

Spirituality partly consists of our beliefs. Take a moment and think about that. What do you believe in? Do you believe in the capacity to heal, or do you believe you are stuck and can't heal, or that your body has let you down?

---

16 *Online Etymology Dictionary*, "spiritual (adj.)," accessed MONTH, DAY, YEAR, https://www.etymonline.com/word/spiritual#etymonline_v_24365.

Spirituality also includes our dreams...our creativity, our vision, and our values. So, it goes into the "heart" of the matter.

It includes each individual's purpose and what a meaningful life means for each. That answer probably looks different for each unique person.

Most importantly, spirituality encompasses the ability to love yourself and the relationship you have with yourself that will support you through the darkest days and the most anxious and difficult moments. This is key to your healing.

One of the byproducts of holistic healing is the ability to hold yourself more effectively through your pain. But you also need to get your support needs met by reaching out to your support team. A holistic healing focus will help you learn a healthier internal dialogue and some healthier behavioral patterns. You can start to reset your sensory system by staying with it and letting the brain process and remap it differently. We have to feel it to heal it. If we keep rejecting and running away or trying to get rid of it, it won't work.

> Just because you are healthy on the outside does not mean you are healthy on the inside. Disease manifests itself in one of three places: mind, body, or spirit. But most of the time, it manifests in the spirit first. When the spirit is unhealthy, it often gets unnoticed until a symptom manifests in the mind (anxiety, depression, etc.) or body (disease state).

Remember when I was open and raw with you regarding how you can't fully heal until you heal the mind? Sometimes, when you're stuck, the Spirit will step in to help.

In my case, about a year had passed after I had been diagnosed with HPA-Axis Adrenal Dysfunction, during which I had been doing the prescribed healing regimen. I was feeling so much better—but still not back at 100 percent. I couldn't figure out why. And that's when something really interesting happened.

I can always tell Pappa is trying to catch my attention when He repeats things in threes. It's just our language...our dialect.

I had been praying to Pappa about my concerns that I still wasn't feeling quite 100 percent back to normal, and I asked for His help. Within a week, three different friends mentioned a type of therapy that they thought I needed so that I could address some trauma I had gone through in my late teenage years.

UGH. My stomach ached at the thought of revisiting THAT in my memory that I had so carefully tucked away years ago, never desiring to visit it again. But He had sent me His sign of three...so I obeyed (but I will quickly let it be known I went unwillingly).

To my surprise, it was exactly what I needed.

As I mentioned before, cells hold memory.[17] They have an exquisite ability to sense their environment and respond.[18] Think of a traumatic experience as a virus in our computer encoding system. Unprocessed traumatic memories malfunction our mental and physical processes. These unprocessed memories don't just affect our brain cells; they also affect the body throughout, as it holds that imprint of the traumatic events. The key word here is "HOLDS."

The brain's autonomic nervous system and emotional centers, such as the hypothalamus, play a key role in recovery. Feeling, holding, and nurturing our vulnerabilities as they come up is a bit of an ebb and flow. It's important to learn how to support yourself and work with your emotions instead of pushing them away, or numbing them, or medicating them, or "eating them away," or denying them, or suppressing them. Learning to actually feel through them enables the brain to process them more elegantly. In other words, we need to let go of the "straitjacket" that prevents the nervous system from "shaking it off" and healing.

Mental health therapy can help in unlocking or processing these emotions, which are locked up with the stored trauma, releasing them from being trapped within your cells and in your biochemistry system. They can help you in removing that "straitjacket." When the traumatic

---

17 "Memory," *Evolution News*.

18 Shruti Naik, Nicolas Bouladoux, Johnathan L. Linehan, Seong-Ji Han, Oliver J. Harrison, Christoph Wilhelm, and other contributors, "Commensal-Dendritic-Cell Interaction Specifies a Unique Protective Skin Immune Signature," *Nature* 520 (2015):104–108. https://doi.org/10.1038/nature14052.

memory is reintegrated into the mind, the brain, and therefore the body, can begin to heal.

That's why six months of therapy for my "perfectly tucked away" trauma turned out to be the last, much-needed step of my HPA-Axis Adrenal Dysfunction healing. Until I healed from the trauma, my Mind-Body-Spirit could not fully heal. This is what we mean by "whole-body healing."

> Healing is about more than reconnecting the hipbone to the thighbone to the knee bone; it is about reconnecting to our souls.

Healing and Self-Discovery

The holistic part of Functional Medicine brings a much deeper ability to heal the patient because, as the old saying goes, the whole is truly greater than the sum of its parts. Sometimes, hints about the healing journey truly do come from surprising and unexpected sources, especially when your heart is ready and the hunger for knowledge is there. Whether you call it "synchronicity" or intuition or a higher power that is meant to help you, if you're open to receiving help, it will come in unexpected ways.

The process of healing can also teach you more about yourself. In a way, it is like a journey.

My healing journey felt like I was walking through a dark valley and climbing my way to the mountain top. Some would say there's beauty at the top because you can see far and wide. But while there might be beauty to see on top, I believe the climb to reach it is more beautiful because it is filled with spiritual growth and less "self-dependency."

When I was ill and trying to rest, I was alone a lot, spending lots of time with Pappa. I felt every emotion—anger, frustration, confusion, crying—because life was NOT as it used to be. The rug was pulled out from underneath me.

The spiritual awakening was just as profound as the physical healing. We don't always truly realize the false identities we pick up throughout our lives and the false agreements we make that rob us of our joy.

When I, the hard-core workout girl, could no longer work out, who was I?

The old, expected reply, "Of course I can do that," slowly transformed into that peaceful "No, I will pass, but thank you." I was finally making space for me.

The formerly extraverted woman who had to be at every gathering, party, event, etc., started appreciating the introvert ways of retreating to find peace within.

The juggling of twelve balls at one time immediately decreased to working with only one.

> In this quiet season of healing, I came to realize that I had been living my life for years trying to carry out those lies I took on myself as truth—living on the go, "fast and furious," trying to be superwoman and supermom, never sitting still, taking on anything that came my way and doing it at 110 percent ... never wanting to disappoint anyone.

My healing journey felt as if it were a time of rebirth for me in all areas of Mind-Body-Spirit. I grew. **I grew in knowledge of how we are tightly woven as Mind-Body-Spirit tapestries**, something my conventional medicine training never mentioned. **I grew in my relationship with the Lord**, which became stronger and deeper and grew out of the false identity I somehow picked up on the way. **I grew in my knowledge of biochemistry and science**, constantly reading evidence-based studies of natural healing. My eyes were opened to a larger scope of healing modalities much different than the approaches my conventional medicine training explored. Don't get me wrong, my conventional training laid the foundation for my purpose, and I use it daily in helping my clients. But I integrate it with Functional Medicine, just like all the other MDs, NPs, and NDs in my peer group at the Institute of Functional Medicine and the School of Applied Functional Medicine.

Tips for Listening to Your "Guiding Power"

The times in my life when I feel the driest in my soul are the times I feel the farthest away from Pappa. They're also times I have been so busy that I haven't slowed down enough to pay attention to my own thoughts, feelings, and emotions. This typically ends up with me finding myself in a striving instead of thriving lifestyle.

When I do slow down and listen, I tune back into intuition. For instance, I spend time in nature, prayer, yoga, meditation, or conversation with Pappa. (Yes, I do talk out loud to Him. I also carry on a conversation in my head with Him...any way I can find to connect with Him to thank Him, praise Him, show gratitude, or even ask for guidance). Then, I become more discerning and aware, taking my thoughts captive then letting go of those thoughts that are not meant to be mine. I also become a better listener for not just myself but a better listener of others. Some call this intuition from a "Higher Power." I personally call it the Holy Spirit.

> "I heard you speak at a conference and it really opened my eyes. It's crazy, because I had just prayed that morning for some guidance on my health—the first prayer I had done in several years. Then there you were, just four hours later on stage speaking as if you were speaking straight to me. I don't believe this to be just coincidence. So, I've taken in every word you said and started incorporating that into what you called a 'lifestyle change' .... My next step is to recheck my labs next week, then I am coming to you for a consultation because I'm ready to be completely 100 percent healthy." —*Tasha, Missouri*

A New Script

You might have a relationship with Pappa too. He may have your heart, but friend, He does not have your fork. That part is up to you.

I've mentioned nutrition in every chapter in this book because it is your MAIN foundation element for good health. If you are putting unhealthful things into your body, it shouldn't be a surprise that you aren't feeling healthy. So, it makes sense to make changes in this area, not just for inflammation but for all kinds of good results.

But the same thing is also true for the nourishment you are giving your mind and spirit. If you are not nourishing your full Mind-Body-Spirit completely, the results will eventually show themselves. Functional Medicine truly does require that you think of all these aspects as equally important. This is not just a new script for the food you cook in your kitchen and put in your body. It is a new script for thinking about your life in a completely different way that will support your health on all levels.

You can have a new birth...a new mindset...a new perspective...a new healthy body...but ONLY after going through the hard labor and delivery of that "birth." You can't just magically make it happen without changing what you yourself are doing. It takes work—every birth requires "labor," right? But it's worth it. And since I've been right there in your shoes, let me walk through the hard parts along with you.

The fresh page is here for turning. The next chapter of your life is waiting to be written. It's your time to shine.

You. Are. Worth. It.

Think of this not only as a new script for your life, but as a new prescription for healing—one that will truly help lead you from Symptoms to Solutions.

CHAPTER 12

Get the Most from Your Consultation

What Next?

If you're going through some major issues (and even if you aren't), it's always better to have a trained practitioner keeping an eye on you. It's easier when you have help figuring out what's really at the heart—or rather, the root—of your symptoms.

And that's where I come in.

My Areas of Specialty

Besides my love for speaking engagements, I have mentioned helping people with the following diagnoses and symptoms that contribute to one or many of these diagnoses in almost every chapter:

Diabetes and Metabolic Syndrome	HPA-Axis Issues
Gut Issues and Reflux	Inflammation
Weight Loss	Heart Disease
PCOS	Adrenal Issues
Thyroid Issues	Sex Hormones Issues
Migraines	Chronic Fatigue

Please know that the mind and spirit affect the body systems. So, from a Functional Medicine perspective, when I address the body-related aspect of the diseases above, I'm also addressing what my client can do for healing of the mind and spirit. There is never a one-size-fits-all approach. Sometimes I have to collaborate/partner with a mental health therapist or a PCP, endocrinologist, cardiologist, or even a psychiatrist, to help my—our—client heal as a whole. Remember, I'm not competing; I'm collaborating for the benefit of the client.

> "Everyone is asking me what I have been doing. They noticed my face was thinning and my clothes were getting baggier! THAT just confirmed even more that your plan works—and it gave me the drive to keep on doing it!" —*Lisa, Arkansas*

What You Can Expect from Treatment

Here's my promise to you:

- **I am your coach, guide, and accountability person.**
  My passion is to unlock your potential to maximize your efforts. As the old Chinese proverb says, "Give a man a fish, you feed him for a day. Teach a man to fish, and you feed him for a lifetime." I desire to teach you how to "fish" so that you are equipped with knowledge and with an internal feeling of, "I got this!" I'm with you every step of the way...including celebrating with you at the finish line!

- **I am your resource for nutrition when you are confused about it.**
  There's so much confusion on the Internet, and I'm here to help you set that straight. You will leave with a meal plan catered specifically to you. These meal plans are centered on nutrient density from phytonutrients, vitamins, and minerals, and they come with recipes that can be modified to even please the tastebuds of the rest of your family.

- **My passion is to help you rebalance your body systems so you can wean off expensive handfuls of prescription medications.**
  Now, I will never tell you to get off a medication; however, I will

most likely recommend you go back to your PCP and discuss the need for weaning AFTER you have been on the healing regimen and have had lots of progress. As the body heals, most people don't need the meds anymore. It really all depends on your body's biochemistry and how it's responding. Most of my patients have either cut back or are completely off meds for high blood pressure, cholesterol, diabetes, anxiety, sleep, inflammation, depression, etc., within just a few weeks to months.

And most importantly, one of the **biggest advantages I can give you at first is my time**. With over two decades of experience, including my own personal journey, and an hour or two to spend in consultation with you, I CAN pick up on something that the other practitioners might not have had time to pick up in their nine to thirteen-minute session with you. I have the time to look at your symptoms and investigate and address their upstream Mind-Body-Spirit root causes, to take you from Symptoms to Solutions.

You Don't Have to Be Local—I Offer Telemedicine

"But wait," you say. "You're not even in my city! I don't want to have to travel hundreds of miles to see a practitioner!"

The good news is that you don't have to.

Many of my clients not only live out of town but out of state. Of course, they prefer telemedicine treatment. And I'm happy to oblige!

I work with my telemedicine clients in exactly the same ways in which I work with my in-person clients. The only difference is that we use a form of videoconferencing instead of meeting in person. As with each client, I start off with an extended consultation to make sure we both have the right information and understand the next steps to take.

Many times, the client will need to make gradual changes in food intake or supplements. We'll always have to tweak a regimen a little because no two people fit into the same mold, and your response to treatment will be unique. We'll discuss those adjustments during our follow-up appointments. The goal is to go by what your body's chemistry needs.

Sometimes a diagnosis or better understanding of progress requires lab work. I give a list of labs to my telemedicine clients so that they can go to their chosen primary care practitioner to have them done. Sometimes labs aren't needed, or sometimes I just need to mail clients an "at home" test, such as the "DUTCH" (Dried Urine Test for Comprehensive Hormones) test or stool test. I also look for certain physical signs on a person, which I can do easily via video conferencing, with my client using a small mirror to see what I'm talking about. Sometimes clients need to send pictures of a urinalysis strip to me.

I keep any necessary testing as simple as possible. We always schedule follow-up visits, and clients have easy access to contact me at any time during office hours.

"I'm so glad you do telemedicine! I could not find a Functional Medicine practitioner in my area. Oh, and by the way, no more stomach pains and rashes! I've stuck to the plan you made out for me, with the exception of being more relaxed on vacation about it, and my twenty-plus years of stomach issues are now resolved. I'm telling everyone about you!" —*Stephanie, Tennessee*

Planning Your First Visit

Prepare to spend some good upfront time—one-and-a-half to two hours, in fact—with me on the first visit.

I really like to take time to get to know you and what has led you to your current health situation, and I just can't get to the root cause of your issues if I am under time constraints like PCPs in insurance. But I team up with PCPs to help out in the process to heal you.

Also, you'll want to have an idea of what you want to get out of your visit and how I can best help you as an individual, so we can discuss that in the initial consultation. For instance, some people know they want a program where they can count on follow-ups regularly, so they feel accountable to someone, as I mentioned. But other people only want initial consultations and then to either be set free or to have follow-up visits weeks down the road to make minor changes.

We'll determine the route that best fits you and your goals. Remember, I'm here to support and help you, which means I will meet you in whatever mental state you're in.

You should be ready to answer these questions on the Nutrition Intake Form that you get when you book an appointment (hopefully, this should be a piece of cake after reading this book!):

What's the most important health issue you want to address?

_____

When was the last time you felt well?

_____

Did something trigger your change in health?

_____

What makes you feel better?

_____

What makes you feel worse?

_____

How does your condition affect you?

_____

What do you think is happening and why?

_____

What do you feel needs to happen for you to get better?

_____

How confident are you in your ability to follow through with this on your own, or are there any aspects of yourself or your life that lead you to question your capacity to do so?

_____

What is your motivation? What is your "why"?

_____

How much accountability do you think you need to help you reach your health goals?

_____

What to Have Before We Start

If you have had any lab work done (blood, stool, urine, saliva, etc.) in the last six or so months, please send those results in with your Intake Form (accessed from my website at www.ChristieBrooksRD.com). This will jump-start the legwork on assessing which routes we need to take for the next step!

When You're Ready to Get Started

Let me see your sweet face! I'm so excited to get to walk alongside you on this new health journey! Here's the process:

Step 1: Set up your appointment accessed on my website. www.ChristieBrooksRD.com

Step 2: Pay either the deposit or the full amount. Your deposit holds your appointment, and it will be deducted from your cost of the initial appointment.

Step 3: You will get a confirmation email and/or text with a Nutrition Intake Form for you to DOWNLOAD onto your computer IN YOUR NAME. Complete it in as much detail as possible. This MUST be turned in (via email ChristieBrooksRD@gmail.com, snail mail, or dropping by the office if you're local) so that I have it at least two days before your booked appointment.

Step 4: Turn in any extra lab work you have had done in the last six or so months when you turn in your Nutrition Intake Form.

Step 5: Come to your appointment in anticipation of receiving a unique healing plan created just for you.

I look forward to meeting you—and get ready to regain your health!

Thank You

Thank you for taking the time to let me guide you through a little bit of the Functional Medicine process and how it might help you. If my experience can help at least one person in a thousand, then I've still accomplished my purpose and what my heart has set out to do...which is to help and heal.

If any part of this book has hit home with you or if you immediately thought of someone who could benefit from reading it, by all means, share this book or tell them about it.

And as I mentioned, I've just grazed the surface here. Your health is highly individualized, and I can only skim the surface in these few pages. This is why I love meeting with people one-on-one, whether in person or via telemedicine. And whether or not we do have the chance to meet, I wish you success on your own health journey, and I hope this book has helped lead you in the right direction toward the best solutions for you.

Acknowledgments

This book is a distillation of stories and lessons I learned during more than twenty-five years of educated work, client interactions, and my own personal healing journey.

It is only possible because of Pappa, who kept opening the doors every time I hungered and thirsted for more knowledge to overcome either my own trials or my clients' challenges during their healing journeys.

A thanks to my OBGYN, TJ Moix, for being vulnerable and directing me towards answers outside of her conventional medicine training, based on those she had found in her own search for real solutions.

A big thank you to my husband, Ashley, for being the anchor and supporting my thirst for knowledge through the years. And thanks to my children, Lexi and Lawson, for their patience when dinner was not ready, or laundry was not quite done because I was buried in science.

A big thanks to my dear yoga, meditation, and/or Ayurvedic friends, Jenny Edwards, Cheryl Weaver, and Kelly Gardner, along with the many others who have journeyed beside me, constantly giving me a feast of research and resources.

A thanks to the mental health therapist I now call friend, Stephanie Marlowe, whom the Lord used to open my eyes on how stored trauma affects the body.

A thanks to the Institute of Functional Medicine (IFM) and the School of Applied Functional Medicine (SAFM) for helping put the pieces of the puzzle together for me to grasp, digest, and apply so that I can help those clients that the Lord puts in my path.

A thanks to all the PCPs, NPs, PAs, specialists, mental health therapists, chiropractors, and trauma yogis that have trusted me to collaborate with them in helping heal shared patients/clients. Thank you for allowing me to be your partner in achieving our clients' whole-body healing. It's an honor.

About the Author

Christie Brooks is a wife to Ashley and a mom to two priority blessings, Lexi and Lawson. Her greatest passion is to help others holistically heal in all areas of Mind-Body-Spirit for a whole-body, root-cause healing. While she has written for numerous magazines, and spoken at a multitude of events, conferences, and for athletic teams over the years, she's best known for her large breakfast feasts after a load of kids have spent the night; love notes in lunches; and her sideline cheerleading at every sports event her children participate in. She loves her family and Pappa passionately and has struggled like everyone else has with stress, too many irons in the fire, laundry, and cellulite.

Symptoms to Solutions

If this book has inspired you, I would love to meet with you in person or telemedicine. Accountability and support are offered and encouraged.

Your journey to better health can start today.

By this time next month, you could be feeling better, moving better, looking better, and starting to see the transformation. You could possibly even be weaning off prescription medications or getting completely off them if your doctor sees progress.

Fatigue	Blood Sugar/Diabetes
Chronic Fatigue	Cholesterol/Blood Pressure/
Low Sex Drive	Heart Disease
Heavy Periods	Inflammation
Adrenal Dysfunction	Fibromyalgia
Thyroid Issues	Stress
Gut/Stomach Issues	Trauma
Sleep Issues	Nervous System Issues
Aches/Pains	Weight Loss
Food Allergy/Intolerances	PLUS MORE!

Includes:

- Initial Functional Medicine Assessment (Plan 1.5-2 hours)
- Analyzation of Health History and Symptoms
- Health Habits Plan
- Lifestyle Plan
- InBody (Muscle-Fat Body Analysis)
- Possible Urinalysis and/or Blood Tests
- Monthly Newsletter (Latest Nutrition News & Recipes)

Book online today for your appointment.

www.ChristieBrooksRD.com

Made in the USA
Las Vegas, NV
13 October 2023

79046892R00079